Superfoods for life

CHIA

Superfoods for life

CHIA

_BOOST STAMINA
_AID WEIGHT LOSS
_IMPROVE DIGESTION
_75 RECIPES

Lauri Boone, R.D.

FAIR WINDS
PRESS
BEVERLY, MASSACHUSETTS

First published in the USA in 2014 by
Fair Winds Press, a member of
Quarto Publishing Group USA Inc.
100 Cummings Center
Suite 406-L
Beverly, MA 01915-6101
www.fairwindspress.com
Visit www.QuarrySPOON.com and help us celebrate
food and culture one spoonful at a time!

18 17 16 15 14   2 3 4 5

ISBN: 978-1-59233-572-5

Digital edition published in 2014
eISBN: 978-1-61058-924-6

Library of Congress Cataloging-in-Publication Data available

Cover design by Paul Burgess
Book design by Kathie Alexander
Photography by Glenn Scott Photography
Additional Photography by shutterstock.com
on pages 13, 44, 76, 102, 105, 135, 144, 163
Styling by Catrine Kelty

Printed and bound in China

The information in this book is for educational purposes only. It is not
intended to replace the advice of a physician or medical practitioner. Please
see your health care provider before beginning any new health program.

Dedication

For Lucky Dog

Chia

Are you ready to bring the power of the chia seed to your plate? Chia is an ancient food that has quickly become a modern-day superstar. A powerhouse of nutrients, chia seeds are packed with minerals like bone-building calcium, stress-busting magnesium, immune system–supporting zinc, and blood-building iron.

They are also one of the richest known plant sources of inflammation-fighting omega-3 fatty acids, and they are bursting with heart-healthy, gut-friendly dietary fiber—which may also hold the key to lasting weight loss. And if you are an athlete (or simply looking to stay active and moving), chia's blend of energy-yielding carbohydrates and high-quality protein will give your body the steady supply of energy it needs to fuel you through exercise, training, and daily life.

Offering a host of beneficial nutrients in a small package that is incredibly simple to work with (and I do mean simple!), the ancient chia seed is shooting to the top of the superfood charts and no wonder. Chia seeds can be easily incorporated, in surprisingly small amounts, into nearly any diet for a powerful boost to health and well-being. And as chia seeds become more readily available in supermarkets and health food stores, nearly everyone—from athletes and executives to yogis and wellness warriors—is scooping up the power of these seeds. In this book, you will learn how to bring the power of chia to your plate—simply and deliciously.

Getting Started: How to Use This Book

Superfoods for Life: Chia is your comprehensive guide to chia seeds. In this book, I combine science-based information on chia and its nutrients with practical tips for incorporating this power food into your own diet. Whether your goal is to lose weight, have more energy, improve digestion, or simply get healthy, you will be armed with the knowledge and know-how of using chia seeds to support your health and wellness goals. What will you find in this book?

- Science-based information on the chia seed and the nutrients within it—after all, knowledge is power. In Chapters 1 through 5, we explore the research on chia and its nutrients as it pertains to issues such as weight loss, athletic performance, digestion, and management of health conditions like heart disease and diabetes. And as you begin to learn more about the incredible health benefits of chia, you will surely be inspired to make it part of your daily or weekly diet.

DID YOU KNOW?

Chia seeds are the edible seeds of an annual, desert-growing plant (*Salvia hispanica*) that is part of the mint (*Lamiaceae*) family and thought to be native to parts of Central America and Mexico. The tiny black and white seeds, which measure only about 1 millimeter in diameter, were a staple food in the diets of the ancient Aztecs and Mayans, who consumed them for increased energy, strength, and stamina. Although chia consumption reportedly declined sometime after the Spanish conquest and fall of the Aztec empire (possibly due to interest in cultivating crops more familiar to the Spanish), it is thought to have begun to increase sometime during the 1900s. A related plant known as golden chia (*Salvia columbariae*) is native to parts of the southwestern United States, and the seeds were thought to be a staple food of Native Americans. However, the chia that is commercially produced today and to which I refer in this book is that of the plant *Salvia hispanica*.

- Practical tips to help you put what you learn into practice. At the end of each chapter you will find a "Putting It into Practice" section, where I provide a concise list of easy-to-implement tips outlining how you might use chia to support your individual goals. Incorporate one, a few, or all of the tips in each chapter to fit your unique diet and lifestyle.

- 75 chia-inspired recipes! After you read about the amazing properties of chia, you may be inspired to create a few of the simple—and delicious—chia-based recipes provided in each chapter. I've got you covered with 75 fast and fun, gluten-free recipes, from refreshing drinks and creamy puddings to savory main courses and sweet treats (plus "Make It Vegan" tips for those who want to create totally plant-based fare). And the best part: The recipes skillfully combine the power of chia with other superfood ingredients to maximize nutrition and taste. Some of my favorite metabolism-boosting, bloat-busting, inflammation-fighting, and beautifying superfoods are incorporated into chia-inspired recipes for nourishment and flavor.

For those of you who simply want to get started start creating chia-inspired dishes in your own kitchen, you can try out any of the recipes in Chapters 1 through 5 or jump ahead to Chapter 6, Chia Seed Essentials: Tips for Working with Chia. In this chapter, I provide the ins and outs of working with chia—from selecting and storing to cooking and baking. And with my flexible recipe templates, you will also learn, step by step, how to create a few staple dishes (like chia gels, puddings, frescas, and no-bake bars)—flavored up your way!

Of course, you can browse the list of FAQs (frequently asked questions) at the back of the book to find answers to some of the most popular questions about chia. (For example, can you eat the chia seeds that came with your Chia Pet?) And if you are looking for additional resources on chia, you can consult the Resources section on page 181.

Whether you want to learn more about the health benefits of chia seeds or begin working with chia seeds in your own kitchen, or perhaps a little of both, this book will be your guide. Are you ready to get started?

Nutrient Data for Chia Seeds (1-Ounce Serving)*

Calories	138 kcals
Carbohydrate	11.9 grams
Total Dietary Fiber	9.8 grams
Protein	4.7 grams
Total Fat	8.7 grams
Saturated Fat	0.9 grams
Monounsaturated Fat	0.7 grams
Polyunsaturated Fat	6.7 grams
Cholesterol	0 milligrams

Minerals

Calcium	179 milligrams
Iron	2.2 milligrams
Magnesium	95 milligrams
Phosphorous	244 milligrams
Potassium	115 milligrams
Sodium	5 milligrams
Zinc	1.3 milligrams

Vitamins

Vitamin C	0.5 milligrams
Thiamin	0.2 milligrams
Riboflavin	0.05 milligrams
Niacin	2.5 milligrams
Vitamin B12	0 milligrams
Vitamin A	15 International Units (IUs)
Vitamin E	0.1 milligrams

*1 ounce (28.35 g) is equivalent to about 2 to 2½ tablespoons of chia seeds.

SOURCE: USDA NATIONAL NUTRIENT DATABASE FOR STANDARD REFERENCE, RELEASE 25. HTTP://NDB.NAL.USDA.GOV/

CHAPTER 1

Fiber-Rich Chia For a Healthy Weight

The tiny chia seed is an ideal power food to help you lose weight. Chia seeds are packed with inflammation- and fat-fighting antioxidants and omega-3 fatty acids; a balanced blend of energy-balancing carbohydrates and protein; weight-supportive minerals like calcium; and satiating dietary fiber—all of which contribute to its ability to help you lose weight. The protein and fiber in chia balance your blood sugar and make you feel sated while its healthy dose of minerals support your digestion and metabolism.

Adding just a small amount of these super seeds to your daily diet may help reduce your appetite, curb cravings, and keep you feeling fuller longer—so you eat less. And as you will discover in the next chapter, chia seeds also provide your body with a steady supply of energy to help keep you active and moving—not crashing and burning. As a result, you will have the vigor to embark on longer and more intense calorie-and fat-blasting workouts and the metabolic boost your body needs to shed (and keep off) those pesky pounds. Indeed, chia seeds are an incredibly simple and effective addition to the weight-loss toolbox of nearly anyone trying to achieve and maintain a healthy weight.

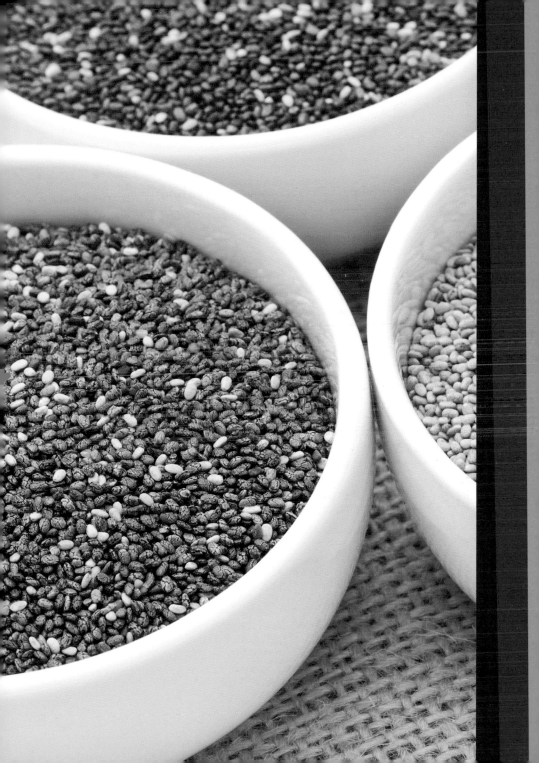

SUPERFOODS FOR WEIGHT LOSS

Can a single food like chia really help you lose weight? Negative energy balance (consuming fewer calories than you expend) is probably the most important factor affecting how much and how quickly you will lose weight, so there is no underestimating the power of eating less and moving more. However, weight loss is far more complex than a simple mathematical equation of calories in and calories out—so yes, certain foods like chia seeds may help support your weight loss efforts.

When I began researching and writing my first book, *Powerful Plant-Based Superfoods* (Fair Winds Press, 2013), I discovered that there were several foods whose properties or combination of nutrients can affect weight. From the fat-blasting potential of super fruits like mangosteen and maqui berries to the metabolism-boosting power of green tea and cayenne pepper, foods (and the nutrients within them) are a powerful weapon in the battle of the bulge.

As you explore the recipe section in this chapter, you will find that I have combined chia seeds with several other food superstars to create a variety of sweet and savory recipes to help maximize your weight-loss efforts. And unlike processed "diet foods"—you know, meal-replacement shakes, bars, and snacks—these whole food, superfood dishes will help nourish your body with their naturally high levels of nutrients that are needed for optimal weight and health—helping you look better and feel better!

High-Fiber Diets Linked to Lower Body Weights

When it comes to supporting weight loss, the magic of the nutrient-dense chia seed lies in its remarkable levels of dietary fiber. Experts agree that fiber is a key factor in achieving a healthy weight—and chia seeds are packed with plenty of it. A single ounce (28.35 g) of chia seeds (about 2 to 2½ tablespoons) contains nearly 10 grams of dietary fiber—30 to 40 percent of your daily needs. And that fiber does much more than keep your digestive tract functioning optimally; it may also help you lose weight.

Studies have shown that high-fiber diets are linked to lower body weights, plain and simple. By contrast, high-fat, low-fiber diets have been linked with an increased risk of being overweight or obese. And the unfortunate news is that most people's diets are too low in fiber. In fact, experts estimate that the average American consumes only about 15 grams of dietary fiber each day, far below the recommended intake of 25 to 35 grams for health. But here's the good news: The simple action of increasing fiber in your diet—with a little boost from chia—may help you reach and maintain a healthy weight.

In a study published in the *American Journal of Clinical Nutrition* in 2003, researchers examined the dietary patterns of thousands of women over a 12-year period. They found that although many women gain weight as they age, those who consume more dietary fiber and whole grains consistently weigh less than those who consume less fiber and whole grains (and subsequently more refined grains). Researchers estimated that an extra 12 grams of dietary fiber per day led to about 8 pounds (3.6 kilograms) less weight gain over the 12 years that the women were followed. And that is the amount you find in just more than 1 ounce (2 to 2½ tablespoons) of chia seeds.

Fiber-Rich Chia Seeds (Literally) Fills You Up

You already know that high-fiber diets are linked with lower body weights. And according to the Academy of Nutrition and Dietetics, consuming 20 to 27 grams of fiber from whole foods each day may help you lose weight and improve your health. Just a tablespoon or two (12.5 to 25 grams) of chia seeds added to your daily diet can provide the additional 10 grams of dietary fiber that most diets are lacking. So how, exactly, do fiber-rich chia seeds work their magic when it comes to weight loss?

High-fiber foods like chia add bulk and volume to meals and snacks to help keep you full; slow digestion and gastric emptying (the rate at which food begins to pass from the stomach into the small intestine); and reduce the release of sugar into the bloodstream (supplying you with a steady stream of energy). Together, these actions help promote satiety, decrease subsequent hunger and cravings, and help you feel fuller longer and eat less—important factors in weight loss.

In a small-scale, randomized, double-blind, placebo-controlled study published in 2010 in the *European Journal of Clinical Nutrition*, researchers looked at the effects of consuming a chia-enriched white bread on the blood sugar levels and appetites of 11 healthy participants. In the study, subjects consumed white bread baked with either 0, 7, 15, or 24 grams (up to a maximum of about 2 tablespoons) of milled chia. Not only did researchers notice a dose-dependent reduction in blood sugars after subjects ate the chia-enriched bread (meaning the more chia baked into the bread, the lower their blood sugars after consuming it), but participants also reported reduced appetites within 2 hours of consuming the chia-enriched bread. And the more chia the bread contained—again, up to about 2 tablespoons (25 grams) providing nearly 10 grams of dietary fiber—the sooner the subjects' appetites decreased.

Because fiber helps you feel full, keeping your hunger at bay, consuming fiber-rich foods like chia may help you eat less and subsequently lose weight. But you may be wondering how much fiber you need to consume at a single meal to experience such effects. Researchers have found that consuming 10 or more grams of dietary fiber at a single meal or snack may help promote satiety (less than that seems to have little immediate effect). And over the long term, regardless of how many calories you consume each day, an extra 14 grams of fiber added to your daily diet appears to reduce the total number of calories you consume by 10 percent, with a potential weight loss of about 4 pounds (1.8 kilograms) over a 3- to 4-month period. These are fairly impressive findings if you consider that you can potentially lose about 12 pounds (5.4 kilograms) a year simply by adding a little more fiber to your diet each day.

 DID YOU KNOW?

Chia seeds are hydrophilic. They have the ability to literally "soak up" the liquid into which they are placed, expanding about 9 to 10 times their actual weight in water. As a result, chia seeds are ideal for thickening beverages and creating puddings and gels, the latter of which can be used as an egg replacer in baking (see Chapter 6 for more information). The remarkable "swelling" action of the chia seed also helps you feel full. It is thought that chia seeds not only swell when placed in liquid, but also in your stomach where they add volume and help slow digestion—an added bonus for those looking to lose weight.

Tiny Seeds with Powerful
Weight-Loss Supporting Nutrients

In addition to its rich content of dietary fiber, chia also contains other nutrients that may play a role in weight loss. Chia seeds contain about 2 grams of high-quality protein per tablespoon (12.5 g). And like fiber, the addition of protein to a meal or snack helps increase satiety, even more than the addition of dietary fat. As a result, the protein from chia seeds also helps keep hunger at bay, gives you a steady supply of energy by slowing the release of sugar into the bloodstream, and leaves you feeling fuller and more satisfied longer.

Chia seeds are also a rich source of the inflammation-fighting omega-3 fatty acid known as alpha-linolenic acid (ALA), which may have a positive impact on both weight and health. In a study published in 2009 in *Nutrition Research*, researchers failed to find any significant changes in the weight and body composition of a small group of overweight or obese men and women who consumed 50 grams (¼ cup) of chia seeds daily for 12 weeks (one of the only published studies I found looking at the direct effect of chia seed consumption on weight). However, at the end of the study, researchers did find that subjects consuming chia had higher levels of ALA. And other studies have found that ALA, like other plant-based oils (including the monounsaturated fats in olive oil), may help enhance weight loss and improve cardiovascular health—especially in those who are overweight and who have metabolic syndrome (a group of risk factors that raises your risk for heart disease, diabetes, stroke, and other health problems)—when consumed as part of a low-calorie diet.

In animal studies, researchers have found that ALA-rich diets tend to decrease body weight. In a study published in 2002, researchers from the University of Arizona, Tucson, found that the weight of chickens fed a 10 or 20 percent chia-enriched diet was significantly lower than those on the control diet—with losses ranging from 5 percent to more than 6 percent. The meat of chickens fed the chia-enriched diet also contained less saturated fat and higher levels of ALA compared to the meat of those on the control diet.

SPOTLIGHT: WHOLE GRAINS

You can boost your intake of dietary fiber by consuming more fruits, vegetables, legumes (beans, peas, and lentils), and whole grains. (See the table on page 20 for a comparison of the dietary fiber content in these commonly consumed plant foods.) But what exactly are whole grains? According to the Whole Grains Council, whole grains are grains that contain all parts of the grain seed (including the bran, endosperm, and germ) and their naturally occurring nutrients. Whole grain consumption has been associated with improved weight and reduced risk of certain chronic and age-related diseases like heart disease, stroke, and type 2 diabetes.

Whole grains include oats; wheat berries, spelt, farro, and Kamut; wild and brown rice; and naturally gluten-free "pseudograins" like amaranth, quinoa, and buckwheat, which are not technically classified as grains but are prepared and eaten in a manner similar to true grains. Chia seeds are not considered whole grains, but because they are a rich source of fiber and other key nutrients, they may confer some of the same benefits of whole grains, including improved weight and reduced risk of certain diseases. As you explore the recipes in this chapter—and throughout this book—you will find that I have combined the power of whole grains and chia seeds into protein- and fiber-packed dishes to support your health and weight.

Dietary Fiber Content of Various Plant Foods

Do you want to add an extra 12 to 14 grams of fiber to your diet each day to support your weight loss efforts—and digestion and health? You can bump up your fiber intake (and easily meet the overall recommended intake of 25 to 35 grams of dietary fiber per day) by consuming a variety of nutrient-dense, fiber-rich foods. Whole grains, pseudograins, fruits, vegetables, legumes, and nuts and seeds—including just a small amount of fiber-packed chia seeds—are all excellent choices!

Lentils, cooked, 1 cup (198 g), 15.6 grams

Black beans, cooked, 1 cup (172 g), 15 grams

Chia seeds, whole, 1 ounce (2 to 2½ tablespoons [28.35 g]), 9.8 grams

Green peas, raw, 1 cup (150 g), 7.4 grams

Flaxseeds, whole, 2 tablespoons (24 g), 5.6 grams

Quinoa, cooked, 1 cup (185 g), 5.2 grams

Apple, raw, with skin, 1 medium, 4.4 grams

Sweet potato, baked in skin, 1 medium, 3.8 grams

Blueberries, raw, 1 cup (145 g), 3.6 grams

Almonds, whole, 1 ounce (28 g or about 23 whole kernels), 3.5 grams

Brown rice, long grain, cooked, 1 cup (195 g), 3.5 grams

Walnuts, English, 1 ounce (28 g or 14 halves), 1.9 grams

Romaine lettuce, 1 cup (47 g) shredded, 1 gram

SOURCE: USDA NATIONAL NUTRIENT DATABASE FOR STANDARD REFERENCE, RELEASE 25. HTTP://NDB.NAL.USDA.GOV/

In a more recent study published in the *British Journal of Nutrition*, researchers found that when chia was added to a sucrose (sugar)-rich diet in rats, it not only had a positive effect on blood lipid levels (like cholesterol and triglycerides) and insulin resistance, but it also reduced their visceral fat (the abdominal fat that surrounds the organs and is associated with increased risk of certain chronic diseases in humans, like heart disease and diabetes). And although all rats consumed the same number of calories and gained weight, those whose diets were enriched with chia gained slightly less weight during the final two months of the study than those consuming the sucrose-rich diet alone. Indeed, more studies are needed (particularly in humans) to examine the effects of fiber- and ALA-rich chia seeds on weight.

Chia seeds are also an excellent source of calcium, which researchers believe may support weight and fat loss. In fact, low calcium intake—lower than the 1000 to 1200 daily milligrams recommended for most adults—appears to be linked to higher body weights. Researchers are unclear about how exactly calcium may influence weight, but some studies suggest that it may help increase both fat burning after mealtime and fat excretion (preventing more fat from being absorbed). In any case, adding chia seeds to your diet can easily help you meet your daily calcium needs for weight and health. In fact, ounce for ounce, these little super seeds contain five times more calcium than milk. Two tablespoons (25 g) of chia seeds provide about 150 milligrams of calcium, rivaling the 276 milligrams found in a single cup (235 ml) of whole milk and meeting 12 to 15 percent of your daily needs. Chia seeds are a good calcium-rich alternative for those following a dairy-free diet.

Putting It into Practice

Chia seeds are one of the simplest fiber-rich foods that you can add to your diet to help reduce appetite, curb cravings, keep you fuller longer, and support your weight-loss efforts. Here are a few simple ways to incorporate chia into your diet for a healthy weight:

- Try incorporating 2 tablespoons (25 grams) of chia seeds into your daily diet to boost your current fiber intake by an additional 10 grams. If you recall, most Americans consume an average of only 15 grams of dietary fiber per day—far below the recommended intake of 25 to 35 grams and still well below the 20 to 27 grams suggested to support a healthy weight. Gradually adding a couple of tablespoons (25 g) of chia seeds to your diet—sprinkled in small amounts throughout the day (a teaspoon here, a teaspoon there)—is a simple way to boost your fiber intake and close that gap.

- Experiment with the chia-inspired recipes in this chapter to naturally boost your fiber intake—and satisfy nearly any craving from sweet to savory. Start your morning with the Creamy Vanilla Chia Pudding (page 30), Almond Chia Pancakes (page 32), or Spicy Citrus & Berry Smoothie (page 28). Enjoy the Hearty Brown Rice Basmati Pilaf (page 37) or Grapefruit & Avocado Salad with Mangosteen Chia Dressing (page 31) for a satiating lunch or dinner. And satisfy your between-meal sweet and salty cravings with snacks like the Easy Baked Chia Kale Chips (page 38), No-Bake Goji Berry Bars (page 42), or Chewy Chia Ginger Macaroons (page 41). The recipes in this chapter are simple, light, and satisfying—and packed with a powerful combination of fiber-rich chia and nourishing superfoods.

- No time to try new recipes? Simply add chia seeds to your favorite dishes at home. Toss a teaspoon (or two) of chia seeds into freshly pressed juices, smoothies, soups, salads, and cereals—no recipes required! Check out Chapter 6 for tips on working with chia.

- Drink plenty of water. Staying hydrated may help support your weight-loss efforts, as our bodies sometimes mistake dehydration for hunger. Adequate water intake may also help ease the digestive upset that sometimes occurs when you start eating more fiber-rich foods. In fact, increasing your fiber intake rapidly (too much, too soon) without simultaneously increasing your water intake may cause constipation, bloating, and abdominal discomfort. You want your body to feel lean, light, and energized, not heavy and swollen. So in addition to gradually boosting your fiber intake with chia seeds, be sure to bump up your water intake, striving to drink at least eight to ten 8-ounce (235 ml) glasses of pure water each day.

DID YOU KNOW?

Breakfast may hold the key to lasting weight loss. The National Weight Control Registry, a database that currently tracks more than 10,000 individuals who have lost at least 30 pounds (about 14 kilograms) and maintained that weight loss for at least one year, found that more than 78 percent of its participants eat breakfast on a regular basis. Eating breakfast helps you to literally "break" your overnight fast and rev up your metabolism, and it may also help you consume fewer calories throughout the day and especially later in the day. Indeed, studies have shown that breakfast eaters tend to eat less and weigh less than those who skip their morning meal.

If you are still not convinced of the benefits of breakfast—or if you are like a few of my clients who used to insist they were actually hungrier throughout the day (and ate more) when they made breakfast part of their routine—then try my breakfast experiment. For one week, eat a small breakfast each morning and note how you feel immediately after and throughout the day. Do you feel satisfied after eating breakfast or are you hungry soon after? You may be surprised to find that after a few days of enjoying a small and satisfying breakfast, you actually eat less throughout the day (and maybe even lose a pound by the end of the week). In addition to the recipes in this chapter, the Rise-N-Shine Smoothie (page 62), Simple Morning Muesli (page 93), and Super Berry Overnight Bowl (page 120) are all great chia-inspired breakfast options that just might give you the energy and staying power you need from your first meal of the day.

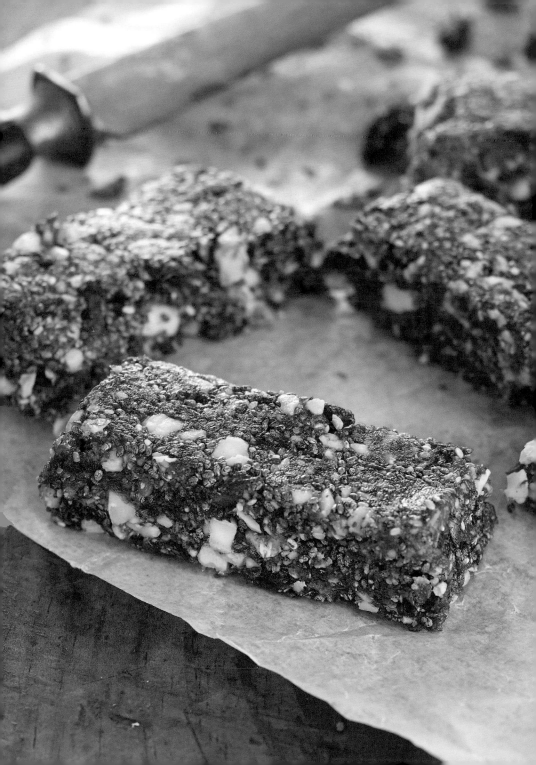

Chia-Inspired Recipes for a Healthy Weight

Fiery Lemon Chia Fresca

This drink is a spicy variation of a traditional lemon chia fresca that relies on a few pinches of cayenne pepper for a fiery kick to wake you up in the morning. Capsaicin, one of the active compounds that gives cayenne pepper its heat, may also give your metabolism a little boost while the vitamin C in lemon juice helps stimulate and support the detoxification pathways of the liver.

2   cups (475 ml) water

3   tablespoons (45 ml) freshly squeezed lemon juice

2   teaspoons chia seeds

1   tablespoon (20 g) pure maple syrup

Few pinches of cayenne pepper, to taste

Combine the water, lemon juice, chia seeds, and maple syrup in a jar with a tight-fitting lid (I like to use a mason jar) and shake to combine. Let stand for about 10 minutes, shaking once or twice.

Pour into a glass, add a few pinches of cayenne pepper, and serve. Refrigerate any unused portion in an airtight container for 2 to 3 days.

Yield: Serves 1 to 2

Pomegranate & Green Tea Chia Fresca

A dynamic duo in flavor and health, green tea and pomegranates are antioxidant powerhouses that are good for the heart—and the waistline. In fact, researchers have found that the catechins in green tea may give metabolism a modest boost while helping to decrease body weight and fat. In this recipe, I like to combine 100-percent pure pomegranate juice with jasmine pearl green tea, which is less bitter and subtly sweeter in flavor than other green teas. But feel free to brew any of your favorite loose leaf or bagged green teas for this refreshing—and nutrient-packed—beverage.

1½ cups (355 ml) brewed jasmine green tea, chilled

½ cup (120 ml) pure pomegranate juice

1 teaspoon freshly squeezed lime juice

2 teaspoons chia seeds

Honey, to taste (optional)

Combine the brewed and chilled green tea, pomegranate juice, lime juice, chia seeds, and honey in a tightly-lidded jar (I like to use a mason jar) and shake to combine. Let stand for about 10 minutes, shaking once or twice. This is best served chilled. Refrigerate any unused portion in an airtight container for 2 to 3 days.

Yield: Serves 1 to 2

Spicy Citrus & Berry Smoothie

Freshly-pressed sweet orange juice combines with the metabolism-boosting and fat-burning power of pure mangosteen juice and coconut oil—two of my favorite "slimming" foods. The addition of fiber-rich chia seeds and raspberries (one of the most fiber-rich of all berries with about 8 grams of fiber per cup [125 g]) will awaken your digestion, while cayenne pepper, a super spice that also seems to act as a natural appetite suppressant, will rouse your tastebuds and kickstart your metabolism.

1½ cups 9355 ml) freshly squeezed orange juice
¼   cup (60 ml) pure mangosteen juice
1½ cups (375 g) frozen red raspberries
1½ cups (375 g) frozen peach slices
1   tablespoon (12.5 g) chia seeds
1   tablespoon (15 ml) coconut oil, melted
    Few pinches of cayenne pepper, to taste

Combine all ingredients (except cayenne pepper) in a high-speed blender and blend until smooth. Pour into one or two glasses, sprinkle with a few pinches of cayenne pepper, and serve.

Yield: Serves 1 to 2

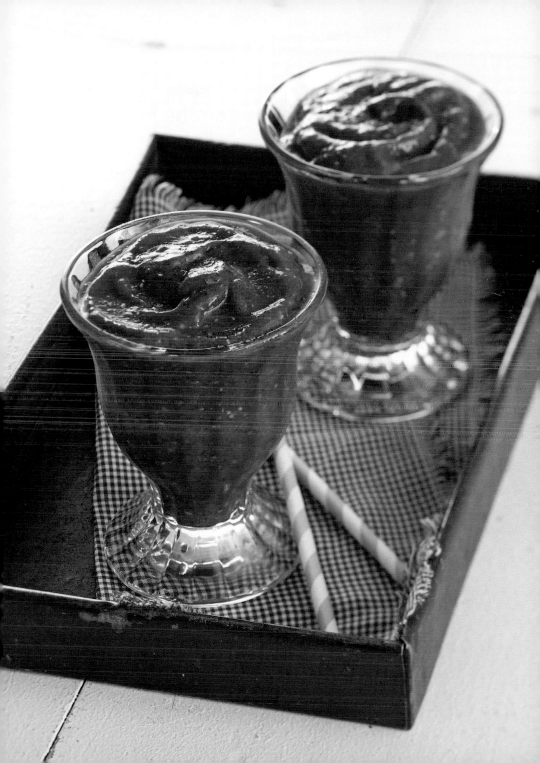

Creamy Vanilla Chia Pudding

Chia puddings are great for breakfast, snack time, or any time—
and deliver a big boost of satiating dietary fiber. In fact, one serving
of this fiber-rich pudding delivers about 10 grams of dietary fiber
from both the chia seeds and the naturally sweet dates. I like to use
thick and creamy unsweetened coconut milk in my chia puddings,
but feel free to use your favorite milk. Just note that if you choose
a sweetened variety of milk that contains added sugar, you might
want to omit the dates to prevent the pudding from becoming
too sweet.

2   **cups (475 ml) unsweetened coconut milk**

4   **pitted dates**

1½   **teaspoons pure vanilla extract**

½   **vanilla bean, scraped, or additional ½ teaspoon pure vanilla extract**

½   **cup (100 g) chia seeds**

     Pure maple syrup, to taste (optional)

Combine the coconut milk, dates, vanilla extract, and vanilla seeds in a high-speed blender and blend until smooth. Pour into a container with a tight-fitting lid (I like to use a mason jar or Pyrex storage dish), add the chia seeds, and shake. Alternatively, you can pour the liquid into a bowl and stir in the chia seeds to combine. Let the pudding rest for 30 minutes, shaking or stirring every 5 to 10 minutes, until thick.

Pour the pudding into serving bowls, drizzle with maple syrup, and serve.

Yield: Serves 3 or 4

Grapefruit & Avocado Salad with Mangosteen Chia Dressing

This light yet satisfying salad combines several superfoods for weight and health: sweet and tangy slices of grapefruit, which may help reduce insulin spikes after meals and boost weight loss; creamy bites of heart-healthy, antioxidant- and fat-rich avocado (with only 50 calories per serving); and a chia-thickened mangosteen dressing.

For the dressing:

2   tablespoons (28 ml) pure mangosteen juice

1   tablespoon (15 ml) freshly squeezed lemon juice

1   tablespoon (15 ml) extra-virgin olive oil

1½ teaspoons chia seeds

1   teaspoon honey

   Sea salt and freshly ground black pepper, to taste

For the salad:

1   heart of romaine lettuce, chopped

3   pink or red grapefruits, sectioned

1   avocado, halved, pitted, peeled, and chopped

½   cup (60 g) chopped walnuts

To make the dressing: In a small bowl, whisk together the mangosteen and lemon juices, olive oil, chia seeds, honey, sea salt, and freshly ground pepper. Set aside to thicken for about 10 minutes.

To make the salad: In a serving bowl, combine the lettuce, grapefruit sections, avocado, and walnuts. Drizzle with 2 to 3 tablespoons (28 to 45 ml) of the dressing, toss to combine, and serve.

Yield: Serves 3

Almond Chia Pancakes

These fluffy pancakes combine milled chia seeds with delicate, finely ground almond meal for a satiating fiber- and protein-packed breakfast treat. Serve these cakes topped with fresh fruit or drizzled with pure maple syrup. Or add a cup (or more) of seasonal fresh fruit to the pancake batter. My favorite additions are fresh blueberries in the summer and chopped apples in the fall.

1½ cups (204 g) Bob's Red Mill all-purpose gluten-free baking flour

¼ cup (28 g) finely ground almond meal/flour

¼ cup (50 g) milled chia seeds

1 tablespoon (14 g) baking powder

½ teaspoon salt

¼ teaspoon ground cinnamon

1½ cups (355 ml) almond milk

¼ cup (60 ml) canola oil (preferably organic, expeller pressed)

2 large eggs

½ teaspoon pure vanilla extract

¼ teaspoon almond extract

In a medium bowl, stir together the flour, almond meal, chia seeds, baking powder, salt, and cinnamon. In a large bowl, whisk together the milk, oil, eggs, and extracts. Stir the dry ingredients into the wet ingredients until just combined and no clumps remain.

Heat a nonstick or lightly oiled skillet or griddle over medium heat. Drop about ¼ cup (60 ml) of batter onto the griddle for each pancake and cook for 3 to 4 minutes on each side until golden brown. Serve warm.

Yield: About 12 (3- to 4-inch, or 7.5 to 10 cm) pancakes

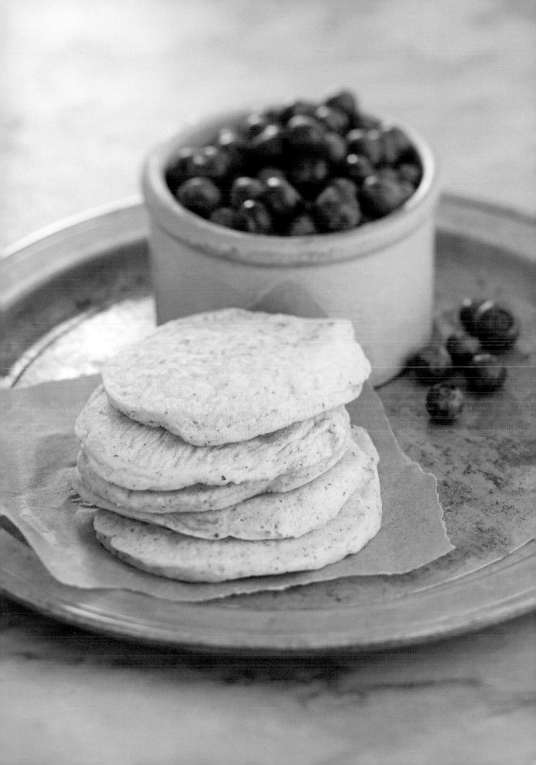

Grilled Asparagus with Balsamic Chia Dressing

Adding a vinegar-based dish, like a salad or vegetable side dish, to a meal is a great way to benefit from the weight-loss-supporting effects of vinegar. Researchers have found that adding vinegar to a meal may increase satiety and slow the rate at which food leaves the stomach (leaving you feeling fuller longer). And studies have found that people who include vinegar at mealtime (typically the morning meal) consume about 200 fewer calories a day than those who do not. Enjoy this dressing drizzled on your favorite grilled or roasted vegetables.

For the dressing:

3   tablespoons (45 ml) extra-virgin olive oil

1   tablespoon (15 ml) balsamic vinegar

1   small clove garlic, crushed

1½ teaspoons chia seeds

1   teaspoon fresh parsley, finely chopped

1   teaspoon fresh basil, cut into thin strips

     Sea salt and freshly ground black pepper, to taste

For the asparagus:

1   pound (455 g) asparagus, tough ends trimmed

     Extra-virgin olive oil, for brushing

     Sea salt and freshly ground black pepper, to taste

To make the dressing: In a small bowl, whisk together the olive oil, vinegar, garlic, chia seeds, parsley, basil, sea salt, and freshly ground pepper. Set aside to thicken for about 10 minutes.

To make the asparagus: Heat a grill pan over medium to medium-high heat. Lay the asparagus in a single layer on the pan. Brush with olive oil and season with sea salt and freshly ground pepper. Grill the asparagus until browned, about 5 minutes. Transfer to a serving platter and drizzle with the dressing. Serve warm or at room temperature.

Yield: Serves 3 or 4

Lemon & Garlic Green Beans

This side dish is simple, light, and flavorful—and it was a staple dish (sans the chia seeds) at nearly every holiday meal when I was growing up. My mom usually topped the mineral-rich green beans with slivered almonds, but I like the added crunch of chia seeds. Serve as a side dish to help you fill at least half of your mealtime plate with vegetables—an ideal strategy for those looking to improve weight and health.

1   pound (455 g) fresh green beans
    (or thawed frozen)

1   tablespoon (12.5 g) chia seeds

1   tablespoon (15 ml) extra-virgin
    olive oil

1   teaspoon freshly squeezed
    lemon juice

1   clove garlic, peeled and quartered
    Sea salt and freshly ground black
    pepper, to taste

Steam the green beans until crisp-tender and bright green, about 5 minutes. Transfer to a serving bowl and toss with the chia seeds, olive oil, lemon juice, and garlic. Let stand for at least 30 minutes to let the beans absorb the garlic flavor.

Remove the garlic pieces (or leave in for a stronger flavor, but do not eat) and season with sea salt and freshly ground pepper. Serve warm or at room temperature.

Yield: Serves 3 or 4

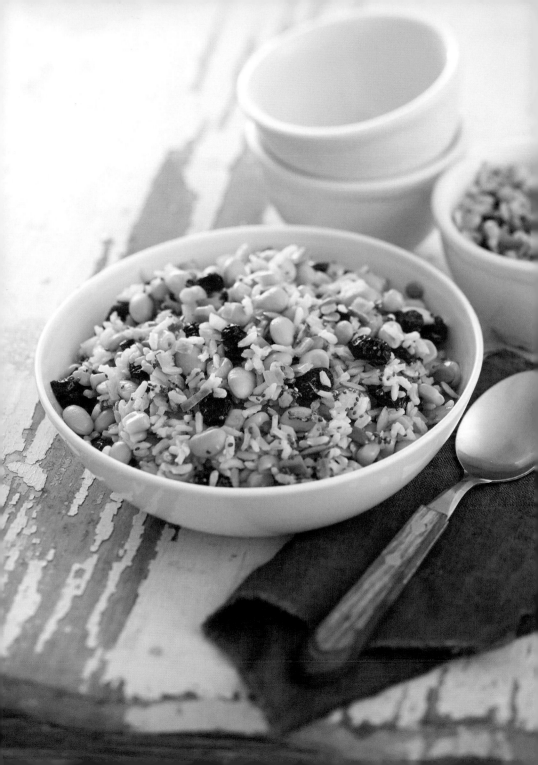

Hearty Brown Basmati Rice Pilaf

This brown rice pilaf is a blend of fragrant whole-grain basmati rice, protein-packed edamame (with more than 17 grams of complete protein per cup), fresh corn, mineral-rich pumpkin seeds, and sweetened dried cranberries—topped off with a few tablespoons (37.5 to 50 g) of chia seeds, of course. Serve as a satisfying fiber- and protein-packed main dish for lunch or dinner.

1   cup (190 g) brown basmati rice

2   cups (475 ml) water

1   tablespoon (15 ml) extra-virgin olive oil

½   medium red onion, finely chopped

2   small cloves garlic, crushed

1   cup (150 g) fresh shelled edamame (or thawed frozen)

1   cup (154 g) fresh corn kernels (or [164 g] thawed frozen)

1   cup (120 g) sweetened dried cranberries

½   cup (32 g) raw pumpkin seeds

2   tablespoons (25 g) chia seeds
     Sea salt and freshly ground black pepper, to taste

Combine the rice and water in a large pot and bring to a boil. Reduce the heat, cover, and simmer for 40 to 45 minutes until all of the liquid is absorbed.

Heat the oil in a large skillet over medium heat. Sauté the onion and garlic until soft, about 3 minutes. Add the edamame and corn to the skillet and cook for about 5 minutes, stirring occasionally, until warm.

Transfer the rice to a serving bowl and stir in the vegetable mixture. Fold in the cranberries, pumpkin seeds, and chia seeds. Season with sea salt and freshly ground pepper and serve.

Yield: Serves 4 to 6

Easy Baked Chia Kale Chips

Kale, a powerhouse of disease-fighting nutrients, can be eaten raw (blended into smoothies, made into juice, or massaged in a salad), cooked (steamed or wilted), or baked into a chip. This simple-to-make kale snack chip (no dehydrator needed!) will surely satisfy your salty and crunchy cravings.

1 to 2 bunches kale (about 1 pound, or 455 g)

1 tablespoon (15 ml) extra-virgin olive oil

2 teaspoons freshly squeezed lemon juice

¼ teaspoon sea salt

2 tablespoons (25 g) chia seeds

Preheat the oven to 300°F (150°C, or gas mark 2). Remove and discard the tough stems from the kale and cut the leaves into 2- to 3-inch (5 to 7.5 cm) pieces. Place the kale leaves in a large bowl and add the olive oil, lemon juice, and salt. Massage the kale leaves until they start to soften, 2 to 3 minutes. Add the chia seeds and toss until the leaves are well coated with the seeds. Lay the leaves in a single layer on 2 large baking sheets and bake for 15 minutes, flipping the leaves over once halfway through cooking, or until crisp. Let the kale chips cool on the pans and serve. Store leftovers in an airtight container for 2 to 3 days. Avoid storing the chips in plastic bags, as they will soften and crumble.

Yield: About 6 cups (420 g)

Cranberry, Orange & Almond Chia Clusters

This sweet and crunchy treat combines one of my favorite flavor combinations—orange and almond—with the chewy sweetness of sweetened dried cranberries. Enjoy a small handful of this nutritious treat between meals for sustained energy and a boost of healthful nutrients.

¼	cup plus 2 tablespoons (120 g) honey
1	tablespoon (15 ml) freshly squeezed orange juice
1	teaspoon orange zest
½	teaspoon pure vanilla extract
¼	teaspoon almond extract
	Pinch of sea salt
2	cups (290 g) raw almonds (1 cup whole, 1 cup roughly chopped)
¾	cup (90 g) sweetened dried cranberries, chopped
¼	cup (50 g) chia seeds

Preheat the oven to 325°F (170°C, or gas mark 3). In a large bowl, whisk together the honey, orange juice, orange zest, extracts, and sea salt. Stir in the whole and chopped almonds, cranberries, and chia seeds and mix until the nuts are coated well. Transfer to a large baking sheet and bake for 25 to 30 minutes, stirring occasionally, until the nuts turn golden brown. Transfer to a large sheet of parchment paper to cool completely. Store in an airtight container or bag in the refrigerator or freezer.

Yield: About 4 cups (600 g)

Garlicky Chia Hummus

This thick and rich hummus is packed with protein, fiber, and minerals like bone-building and weight-loss-supporting calcium (more than 500 milligrams of calcium from the tahini alone). A few pinches of metabolism-boosting cayenne pepper combined with a generous addition of fat-burning garlic may also help boost your weight-loss efforts (researchers have found that some of the sulfur-containing compounds in garlic may help burn body fat)—and boost flavor. Serve this hummus with fresh vegetable slices or use it as a spread on sandwiches, veggie burgers, or sprouted-grain or gluten-free breads.

2   cups (480 g) canned chickpeas, drained and rinsed

½   cup (120 g) roasted tahini

⅓   cup (80 ml) freshly squeezed lemon juice

¼   cup plus 2 tablespoons (88 ml) extra-virgin olive oil

4 to 6 cloves garlic, crushed

2   tablespoons (25 g) chia seeds

1   teaspoon sea salt, or more to taste
     Few generous pinches of cayenne pepper

Combine all of the ingredients in a food processor and process until smooth, stopping as needed to scrape down the sides. Refrigerate any leftovers for up to 5 days.

Yield: About 2½ cups (750 g)

Chewy Chia Ginger Macaroons

These bite-size raw cookies are the perfect go-to snack when you are craving something sweet and chewy. Raw almonds and chia seeds deliver extra fiber, protein, and beneficial fats—for extra staying power—while freshly grated ginger offers up subtle warmth and flavor. You will need a food dehydrator to make these macaroons.

1   **cup (145 g) raw almonds**
1   **cup (85 g) shredded dried coconut**
¼   **cup (50 g) chia seeds**
     Pinch of sea salt
½   **cup (160 g) agave syrup**
¼   **cup (60 ml) coconut oil, melted**
1   **tablespoon (0 g) grated fresh ginger**
1   **teaspoon pure vanilla extract**

In a food processor, grind the almonds into a fine meal. Combine the almond meal, coconut, chia seeds, and salt in a medium bowl. In a large bowl, whisk together the agave syrup, coconut oil, ginger, and vanilla extract. Add the dry ingredients to the wet ingredients and mix thoroughly.

Drop approximately tablespoon-size (15 g) scoops (I use a #60 scoop) onto dehydrator screens and dehydrate at 105°F (41°C) for about 12 hours. The cookies should be dry to the touch, but soft and chewy.

Remove the warm cookies from the dehydrator and let come to room temperature. Store in an airtight container.

Yield: About 30 cookies

No-Bake Goji Berry Bars

These sweet and chewy squares combine the metabolism-boosting power of goji berries with the natural sugars of dates, the fiber-, protein-, and calcium-packed crunch of raw almonds, and chia seeds. Enjoy this simple-to-make snack at home or on the go.

1½   cups (267 g) pitted dates
¾   cup (109 g) raw almonds
½   cup (100 g) chia seeds
½   cup (45 g) dried goji berries
2   tablespoons (40 g) agave syrup

Line a cutting board with waxed paper. Combine all of the ingredients in a food processor and process into a coarse dough. The dough should stick together when pressed with the fingertips. If the dough feels too dry, add another date or small squeeze of agave syrup and process. If it feels too sticky, add a few more almonds or small scoop of chia seeds and process.

Transfer the dough to the cutting board. Press the dough into a large ball and place on the center of the cutting board. Place a second sheet of waxed paper on top of the dough and flatten with the palm of your hand. Using a rolling pin, roll the dough out (with the waxed paper on top) to a ½-inch-thick (1 cm) rectangle, trimming the edges of the dough if needed. Cut the dough into 1 x 3-inch (2.5 x 7.5 cm) bars and set aside. Repeat the rolling and cutting process until there is no more dough left and you have 12 to 15 bars. Store in an airtight container between layers of waxed paper.

Yield: 12 to 15 bars

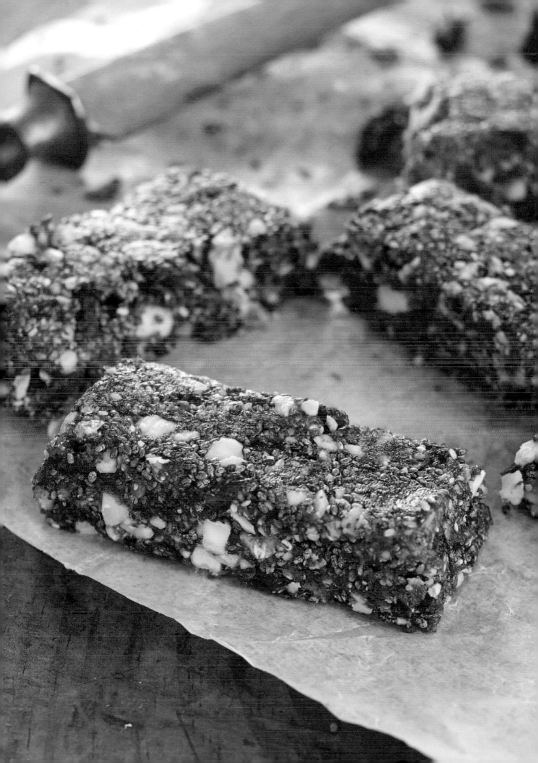

CHAPTER 2

The Super Stamina Seed: Chia for Peak Performance

When I began working with athletes more than a decade ago, I quickly discovered that nearly everyone—from casual and recreational exercisers to elite and professional athletes—wants to not only perform well but also maintain good health. Although many were seeking out ways to be faster, or stronger, or to go longer, they were also frequently struggling with health issues like fatigue, frequent colds and infections (especially following major events like marathons), and digestive upset—issues that affected both their performance and their daily life.

As a sports dietitian, my goal was to help them create a diet to support their training and their health. And that meant teaching them how to easily incorporate the most nutrient-dense whole foods into their diets to give them the biggest bang for their buck—allowing them to be at the top of their game both on and off the field (or track or bike). In recent years, nutrient-rich chia seeds—along with a few other superfoods—have begun to take center stage in the sports kitchen.

Simple-to-Use Runners' Food for Athletes

Chia seeds are an ideal superfood for nearly any athlete or active individual. Their name comes from the Mayan word for "strength," and chia seeds are reported to have been a dietary staple of the Mayans and Aztecs, who used the tiny seeds to help sustain energy levels and increase stamina. And in his book *Born to Run*, author Christopher McDougall reports that the Tarahumara Indians of Mexico consume chia to help fuel them through long-distance runs. Thanks to that book, these power seeds are frequently referred to as "runners' food" and are becoming increasingly popular among athletes, especially those participating in endurance sports.

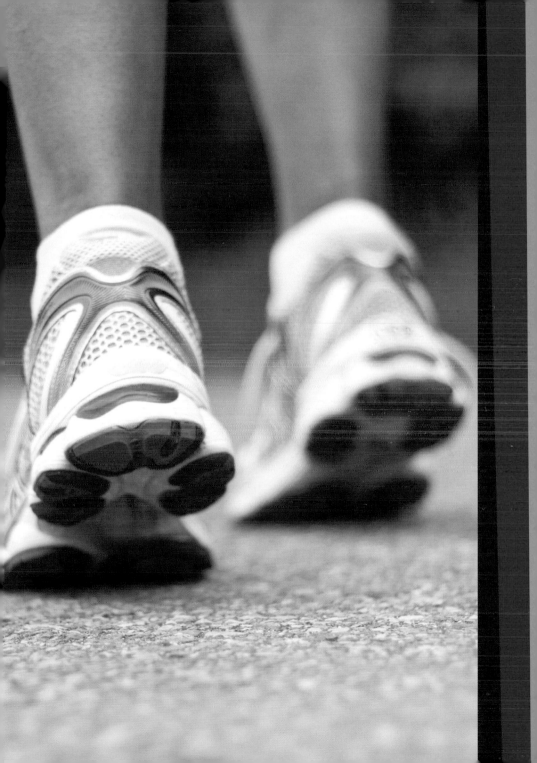

Indeed, chia seeds contain a nice blend of energy-yielding carbohydrate and high-quality, easy-to-digest protein to give your body a steady supply of energy to help keep you active and moving, not crashing and burning. Additionally, chia seeds will not only help give you the energy to perform, but they also contain a rich array of important bone- and blood-building minerals, inflammation-fighting fats, and cell-protecting antioxidants—all of which help nourish the body and counter the stressful effects of intense training and exercise.

Nearly as important as their rich nutrient content—or perhaps even more important for the busy athlete—is the fact that chia seeds are incredibly simple to use and incorporate into the sports diet. Hectic training schedules often afford athletes little time in the kitchen to prepare meals and snacks. As a result, many athletes (and you may be among them) tend to rely on packaged sport and energy bars, boxed cereals, and bottled sports drinks as fuel for daily activity and training. Although these processed foods may provide the calories you need, they tend to offer little real nutrition. Whole foods like chia seeds are a simple-to-use delivery system for the nutrients your body needs to be active and well. From simple-to-blend smoothies to no-bake energy bars, the recipes in this chapter will show you how you can begin to incorporate this super seed into your sports diet with minimal time and the greatest of ease.

Carbohydrate- and Protein-Rich Super Seed for Sustained Energy

Chia seeds contain a nice blend of energy-balancing carbohydrates and protein, and studies have shown that adequate carbohydrate intake is essential to the sports diet, especially for endurance athletes. In fact, researchers have found that consuming too few carbohydrates in the daily diet can actually impair performance and endurance potential—meaning that you won't be able to perform for as long or push quite as hard at the end of your training or event than if your body were well stocked with carbohydrates. And in the event that your body's carbohydrate stores become depleted, you will likely experience "bonking" (sometimes called "hitting the wall"), when your body and brain run out of the crucial fuel from carbohydrates that keep them functioning. So how can you optimize your carbohydrate intake and body stores, how much carbohydrate do you need to consume daily, and how can chia seeds support your training?

The best way to optimize your carbohydrate intake and muscle and liver stores of carbohydrates (called glycogen stores) is to eat a steady supply of carbohydrate-rich foods on a daily basis. Carbohydrate recommendations are highly individual and vary according to your sport and the intensity and duration of your training, among other factors. But in general, researchers recommend that most athletes consume 6 to 10 grams of carbohydrate per kilogram of body weight (2.7 to 4.5 grams of carbohydrate per pound of body weight) daily. For the 150-pound (68 kilogram) athlete, that translates into 405 to 675 grams of carbohydrate each day.

Of course, when I ask athletes to eat a steady supply of carbohydrate-rich foods daily, they usually have one of two opposing reactions: sheer delight or horror at the mistaken idea that I am asking them to fill their plates with bagels, breads, boxed cereals, and pastas. Not so! I encourage them—and you—to skip the empty calories from highly processed foods and instead reach for nutrient-dense whole foods (like chia seeds!) to easily meet daily needs. Whole grains; pseudograins like amaranth and quinoa (see Chapter 1, page 12, for more information on whole grains and pseudograins); starchy vegetables like sweet potatoes, beets, and carrots; legumes (beans, peas, and lentils); a variety of fresh and dried fruits; and even nuts like almonds are all great options. And just a single ounce of chia seeds (2 to 2 ½ tablespoons, or 25 to 31 grams) contains about 12 grams of carbohydrate—the amount you might find in a piece of fresh fruit, a slice of whole grain bread, or a cup (235 ml) of milk.

Researchers have also found that chia seeds can be used effectively in carbohydrate-loading protocols. Carbohydrate loading is a technique that typically involves increasing the amount of carbohydrate in the diet while simultaneously reducing training in the days preceding an event (usually an event that lasts longer than 90 minutes) in order to optimize carbohydrate stores in the body and improve performance. In a small study published in 2011 in the *Journal of Strength and Conditioning Research*, researchers from the University of Alabama at Auburn found that consuming a 50 percent chia–based sports beverage was just as effective for carbohydrate loading—and had similar outcomes on performance in runners—as a traditional sports drink. In addition, the chia-based beverage may benefit athletes who wish to lower sugar intake and increase protein and omega-3 fatty acid intakes—a benefit to health without being a detriment to performance.

Carbohydrate Content Of Various Plant Foods

Athletes can easily meet carbohydrate needs by consuming a variety of whole foods. The carbohydrates found in whole grains, pseudograins, legumes, vegetables, fruits, and even nuts and seeds (like almonds and chia) all contribute to your daily intake.

Brown rice, medium grain, cooked, 1 cup (195 g), 45.8 grams

Chickpeas, cooked, 1 cup (164 g), 45 grams

Lentils, cooked, 1 cup (198 g), 39.9 grams

Quinoa, cooked, 1 cup (185 g), 39.4 grams

Potato, baked with skin, 1 medium, 36.6 grams

Oats, regular or quick, cooked with water, 1 cup (80 g), 28.1 grams

Banana, 1 medium, 27 grams

Sweet potato, baked with skin, 1 medium, 23.6 grams

Raisins, seedless, 1 ounce (28 g or 60 raisins), 22.5 grams

Chia seeds, 1 ounce (28 g), 11.9 grams

Whole wheat bread, commercially prepared, 1 slice, 11.6 grams

Almonds, 1 ounce (28 g or 23 whole kernals), 6.1 grams

SOURCE: USDA NATIONAL NUTRIENT DATABASE FOR STANDARD REFERENCE, RELEASE 25. HTTP://NDB.NAL.USDA.GOV/

High-Quality Protein for Endurance and Strength Athletes

Like carbohydrates, adequate protein in the diet is essential for both strength and endurance athletes. For the endurance athlete, the addition of protein to the diet helps slow the release of sugars into the bloodstream, providing a steady supply of energy for training. And in the presence of adequate calories and carbohydrates, it ensures that amino acids (the building blocks of protein) are used for important muscle and tissue building—not burned for energy, which may occur when you consume too few calories or carbohydrates. Indeed, for both strength and endurance athletes, dietary protein helps support muscle and tissue growth, helps muscles recover from the demands placed on them during training (whether running or lifting weights), and may even help reduce muscle soreness when consumed after exercise. And as you are about to learn, chia seeds offer athletes a simple way to get a small boost of easy-to-digest protein in their sports diet.

Although there is some controversy over whether or not athletes have increased protein needs (it is thought that if an athlete is consuming adequate calories to support training and maintain weight, protein needs will be automatically met), many experts—me included—agree that athletes should be taking in more protein than the 0.8 gram of protein per kilogram of body weight (about 0.4 gram of protein per pound of body weight) recommended for the general population. This is especially true for those looking to lose weight while maintaining lean body mass as well as for those who adhere to strict vegetarian or vegan diets. And every small amount of protein in the diet—including the nearly 5 grams in each ounce of chia seeds—helps you meet your needs.

In general, most research studies support protein intakes of 1.2 to 1.4 grams of protein per kilogram of body weight (0.5 to 0.6 grams of protein per pound of body weight) for endurance athletes and 1.2 to 1.7 grams of protein per kilogram of body weight (0.5 to 0.8 grams of protein per pound of body weight) for strength athletes. For the 150-pound (68 kilogram) athlete, this translates into a wide range of anywhere from 75 to 120 grams of protein per day.

Animal proteins like whey and casein, along with plant-based proteins like soy, are commonly thought of as superior, high-quality, complete protein sources for athletes and non-athletes alike. However, because soy and dairy products are common food allergens, I have found that they are not always well tolerated or easily digested. As athletes start thinking outside the box and look toward alternative sources of easy-to-digest proteins that provide a wide spectrum of amino acids, seeds like chia, hemp, and quinoa have begun to take center stage. With nearly 5 grams of protein per ounce (2 to 2½ tablespoons, or 28.35 g), chia is a simple addition to the diet, and when combined with other protein-rich plant foods like quinoa (a complete protein containing all essential amino acids), hemp seeds (which contain about 5 grams of protein per tablespoon [7.5 g] of hemp powder), whole grains, and legumes provides a full spectrum of all the essential amino acids the body needs.

COMPLETE PROTEINS

Amino acids are the building blocks of protein, and complete proteins contain adequate levels of all nine essential amino acids. The protein in animal products (including meat, poultry, fish, eggs, and dairy products), soy foods (including edamame, tofu, and tempeh), and quinoa are all considered complete. Although chia seeds contain all of the essential amino acids—and are particularly rich in the amino acids arginine and glutamic acid—they are not considered complete, as they have low levels of lysine. However, you can easily meet your protein needs and obtain adequate levels of all the essential amino acids your body needs by consuming a variety of protein-rich plant foods—including chia—over the course of each day. Enjoy a variety of whole grains and pseudograins (like quinoa and amaranth), legumes (beans, peas, and lentils), and nuts and seeds including sacha inchi seeds, hemp seeds, and chia seeds each day—no special combining needed!

Protein Content Of Various Plant And Animal Foods

Athletes (and non-athletes) can easily meet their protein needs by consuming a variety of nutrient-dense, protein-rich foods each day. This table highlights a few popular choices.

Wild Atlantic salmon, 3 ounces (85 g), cooked, dry heat, 21.6 grams

Lentils, cooked, 1 cup (198 g), 17.9 grams

Edamame, prepared, 1 cup (150 g), 16.9 grams

Chickpeas, cooked, 1 cup (164 g), 14.5 grams

Quinoa, cooked, 1 cup (185 g), 8.1 grams

Peanut butter, smooth with salt, 2 tablespoons (32 g), 8 grams

Peas, fresh, 1 cup, (150 g) 7.9 grams

Almond butter, plain with salt, 2 tablespoons (32 g), 6.7 grams

Egg, 1 large, 6.3 grams

Chia seeds, 1 ounce (28 g), 4.7 grams

Multigrain bread, 1 slice, 3.5 grams

SOURCE: USDA NATIONAL NUTRIENT DATABASE FOR STANDARD REFERENCE, RELEASE 25. HTTP://NDB.NAL.USDA.GOV/

Fueling with Chia Before, During, and After Exercise

As you have learned, chia is a nutrient-dense source of carbohydrates and protein in the sports diet. But the nutrient profile of chia seeds also makes them an ideal food that can be easily incorporated into the training diet before, during, and after workouts.

One of the goals of the pre-training meal or snack is to provide easy-to-digest fuel while minimizing stomach upset. In general, pre-training meals should be eaten 3 to 4 hours before exercise and include both carbohydrates and protein to help balance blood sugars and sustain energy levels (sounds like a good fit for chia seeds, right?). Similarly, the post-exercise meal or snack should also consist of both carbohydrates and protein. This meal is intended to help replenish depleted carbohydrate stores, aid in muscle recovery and building, and assist the body in recovering more quickly after exercise and between training sessions (once again, sounds like a good match for chia, right?). Power Muesli (page 65), Lentil and Split Pea Salad with Sacha Inchi Seed Dressing (page 68), and Velvety Banana Chia Pudding (page 64) may serve as ideal meals to help athletes fuel pre-exercise and replenish post-exercise.

Most experts agree that, as you get closer to your workout or event time, you should begin to consume more carbohydrate-rich foods—without the added protein, fiber, and fat that can slow digestion and lead to gastrointestinal distress once you start moving. For this reason, sports drinks, gels, and fruit and fruit juices are commonly recommended within the hour before exercise—and chia seeds, which are a rich source of dietary fiber and omega-3 fats, may not seem particularly ideal. But here's the problem: I have found that these sugar-only foods don't agree with every athlete.

I know from both personal experience and my work with athletes that the pre-exercise snack is highly individualized, depending on the sport, the intensity and duration of training, and the athlete himself or herself. If you are sensitive to sugar, relying on sugar alone may actually make you feel worse when you start exercising. When my pre-run snack consisted of a few simple carbohydrate-rich foods (like a banana, applesauce, or sports drink), I often found myself running with a light head, nausea, and upset stomach. But by adding just a small amount of protein to my pre-run snack, I was able to eliminate those symptoms and maintain my energy levels while I ran. A slice of sprouted-grain bread with a thin spread of almond butter or a banana with a tiny scoop of peanut butter were my stomach-friendly, go-to choices within the hour of my workout. And today, I rely on and recommend a few chia-inspired snacks to provide the carbohydrate—balanced with a small

ONE SPORTS DIET DOES NOT FIT ALL

Just as there is no one diet that fits all, there is no one sports diet (or food) that fits every athlete. In fact, I often say that the best foods for your sports diet are the ones your body tolerates best. If you choose to incorporate chia seeds into your diet, be sure to experiment with this power food during training to discover the optimum amount and delivery method (chia drink, energy bar, or gel?) to sustain your training and leave you feeling good.

Perhaps chia is a perfect day-to-day addition to your sports diet, but not before your morning run. Or maybe consuming chia while exercising upsets your stomach, but you find it's the perfect addition to your pre-training fruit smoothie because the protein keeps you from crashing once your feet hit the pavement. Nutrient-rich chia seeds are worth experimenting with—so experiment freely to discover how you can best incorporate this superfood into your sports and training diet.

amount of protein—to fuel workouts. So if a sugar-only pre-training snack doesn't work for you, you might benefit from tossing a small scoop of chia seeds into your water or sports beverage. Or experiment with a spoonful or two of Velvety Banana Chia Pudding (page 64), a small serving of the Rise-N-Shine Smoothie (page 62), a small square of the Crispy Almond Butter Energy Bars (page 73), or a date-based Chocolate & Maca Chia Chew (page 74) in the hour before you exercise (along with plenty of water, coconut water, or sports drink) to give your body the carbohydrates and small protein boost it may require to feel and perform its best.

The idea of fueling your body during exercise is to provide you with an instant source of energy—namely, carbohydrate—to keep you moving and prevent your body's own carbohydrate stores from becoming depleted. Experts recommend taking in 30 to 60 grams of carbohydrate per hour of exercise from mixed sources including both food (like gels and chews) and beverages (like sports drinks). Although I have found that most individuals fare well by consuming a mix of carbohydrates during exercise (usually a mixture of sugars from sports drinks, gels, broken pieces of sports bars, and energy gel blocks or beans that are consumed during workouts lasting more than an hour), a few others have reported performing better when adding a little protein to the mix. If you are one of those individuals, you may find that adding a small amount of chia seeds to your sports drinks or including a chia-based gel or small portion of a chia-based energy bar provides sustained energy and enhanced stamina. Or you may find that this fiber-rich seed does not sit well in your stomach at all during exercise. In general, I have found that the small addition of protein (typically from nuts and seeds like chia) is most beneficial to those involved in light to moderately intense exercise (think hiking and walking) of long duration.

ANTIOXIDANTS AND MINERALS FOR ATHLETES

Many athletes look toward supplements (protein, amino acid, vitamin and mineral, and herbal supplements) to help meet their energy and nutrient needs. But whole foods—especially superfoods like chia seeds—are naturally rich in nutrients that work synergistically in the body to support both activity and health. Chia seeds are rich in antioxidants, which may help offset the increased production of free radicals that occurs with intense exercise and training. They are also a rich source of alpha-linolenic acid, an omega-3 fatty acid that may help ease inflammation associated with arthritis and joint pain.

In addition, chia seeds are rich in bone-building calcium, which also helps support muscle contraction and nerve conduction. Calcium is one of several minerals (along with iron, zinc, magnesium, and selenium) for which athletes appear to have an increased risk of deficiency. An ounce of chia seeds contains nearly 180 milligrams of calcium (more than the 138 mg in a ½ cup [120 ml] of whole milk), more than 2 grams of blood-building iron (about 10 percent and 25 percent of the recommended intake for most adult men and women, respectively), and about 95 milligrams of stress-relieving magnesium.

Putting It into Practice

Chia seeds are rich in the carbohydrates, amino acids, vitamins and minerals, inflammation-fighting fats, and antioxidants your body needs to keep you performing your best. Here a few simple ways to incorporate chia into your sports and training diet for performance and health:

- To boost your daily intake of high-quality carbohydrates that will keep you active and moving, try adding 1 to 2 tablespoons (12.5 to 25 g) of chia seeds (providing up to about 12 grams of carbohydrate) to your daily diet. Simply toss into your favorite juice, smoothie, salad, or soup.

- In the hour before your workout, try adding a small amount of chia seeds— about 1 teaspoon (more or less) of chia seeds—to water, coconut water, or a sports drink. This may be especially helpful if you are sensitive to sugars and find that you fare better during exercise with the addition of a small amount of protein. If you choose to consume chia pre-exercise, start with a small amount and gradually increase until you find the right amount for balancing blood sugars without upsetting your stomach.

- During exercise, try adding a small amount of chia—about 1 teaspoon (more or less) to your water, coconut water, or sports drink. You can also carry a pre-made Chia Gel (page 166) or small packet of seeds for fuel while you work out; just be sure to follow both up with plenty of water or sports drink. In addition, you can also cut up tiny squares of a chia-based snack like the Spicy Orange & Goji Berry Chia Fruit Leather (page 72), Pomegranate & Lime Chia Fruit Leather (page 156), or any of the no-bake, date-based chia snacks, all of which are easily transported during exercise. As I have previously mentioned, this fueling strategy may be most beneficial to those engaged in lower-intensity exercise of longer duration (like walking or hiking).

- After exercise, consume a chia-based recovery drink like the Gingery Coconut Chia Cooler (page 60) or Superpowered Strawberry & Banana Smoothie (page 61) to help replenish and rehydrate your body. And as you aim to eat within the first 30 minutes after exercise (and ideally every 2 hours for the remaining 4 to 6 hours after exercise), try adding a chia-inspired dish to your meal such as the Creamy Broccoli & Potato Soup (page 66), Lentil and Split Pea Salad with Sacha Inchi Seed Dressing (page 68), or Velvety Banana Chia Pudding (page 64).

- As always, experiment with chia seeds to discover the optimal intake and delivery method that works best for your body and training regimen. Dietary needs and tolerances vary according to athlete, sport, and training protocol.

HYDRATION

I've read some articles stating that chia seeds can help keep you hydrated due to their hydrophilic properties. It's true that chia seeds will soak up and hold onto the fluid in which they are placed, but I'm not sure they can actually help improve hydration status. To stay hydrated, I recommend consuming at least 1 to 2 liters (1 to 2 quarts) of pure water each day in addition to mineral- and electrolyte-rich coconut water, freshly pressed juices and smoothies, and water-rich whole fruits and vegetables. Also be sure to drink fluids during exercise: pure water for exercise lasting 1 hour or less and homemade or commercial sports drink (providing both carbohydrates and electrolytes) for exercise lasting longer than 1 hour. And if you are just beginning to add chia and other fiber-rich foods to your diet, be sure to do so gradually and increase your fluid intake. As I mentioned in Chapter 1, increasing fiber intake too rapidly (especially in the absence of adequate fluids) may lead to constipation, bloating, and abdominal pain—far from a winning combination for athletes.

Chia-Inspired Recipes for Peak Performance

Gingery Coconut Chia Cooler

This invigorating cooler infuses electrolyte-rich coconut water with the inflammation-fighting power of grated fresh ginger. Sometimes called "nature's sports drink," coconut water is a rich source of electrolytes like magnesium and potassium. In fact, 1 cup (235 ml) of coconut water has 600 milligrams of potassium—nearly 150 percent more than a medium banana.

2   **cups (475 ml) coconut water**
1   **teaspoon freshly squeezed lime juice**
¼   **teaspoon grated fresh ginger**
2   **teaspoons chia seeds**
    Honey, to taste (optional)

Combine the coconut water, lime juice, ginger, chia seeds, and honey in a jar with a tight-fitting lid (I like to use a mason jar) and shake to combine. Let stand for about 10 minutes, shaking once or twice.

Serve chilled. Refrigerate any unused portion in an airtight container for 2 to 3 days.

Yield: Serves 1 to 2

SPOTLIGHT: GINGER

Ginger is an inflammation-blocking super spice for athletes. Researchers have found that ginger appears to have the same pain-relieving powers as non-steroidal anti-inflammatory drugs (NSAIDs) like ibuprofen—but without the adverse side effects like stomach upset and ulcers. The active compounds in ginger seem to block the pathways that can lead to the inflammation and pain associated with osteoarthritis and other musculoskeletal conditions. It is so easy to incorporate into your daily sports diet. Simply add fresh ginger to juices and smoothies or sprinkle some freshly grated or dried ground ginger into your favorite soups—for flavor and health!

Superpowered Strawberry & Banana Smoothie

Power up the classic combination of strawberries and bananas with the addition of protein—and fat-rich chia and hemp seeds. This creamy smoothie boasts around 10 grams of protein (more than the 6 grams in a large egg) and has enough iron to meet 10 to 15 percent of your daily needs. And the boost of antioxidant vitamin C from the strawberries and oranges will help your body soak up more of that plant-based iron.

1½ **cups (355 ml) freshly squeezed orange juice**

2 **cups (510 g) frozen strawberries**

1 **medium banana**

1 **tablespoon (7.5 g) hemp seeds**

1 **tablespoon (12.5 g) chia seeds**

Combine all of the ingredients in a high-speed blender and blend until smooth.

Yield: Serves 1 to 2

Rise-N-Shine Smoothie

This sunshine-in-a-glass smoothie offers a beneficial boost of anti-oxidant vitamins A and C from sweet oranges, mangos, and gold-enberries, the latter of which are also packed with energy-yielding B-complex vitamins. A few pinches of turmeric pump up the flavor and the pain- and inflammation-reducing power (curcumin-rich tur-meric may help reduce joint pain and inflammation associated with osteoarthritis) and may even enhance brainpower and mood. This is a great smoothie to kick-start your day—and your workout!

1½ **cups (355 ml) freshly squeezed orange juice**

2 **cups (350 g) frozen mango chunks**

½ **cup (60 g) dried goldenberries**

2 **teaspoons chia seeds**

Few pinches of ground turmeric, to taste

Combine the orange juice, mango, gold-enberries, and chia seeds in a high-speed blender and blend until smooth. Pour into 1 or 2 glasses and sprinkle with a few pinches of turmeric.

Yield: Serves 1 to 2

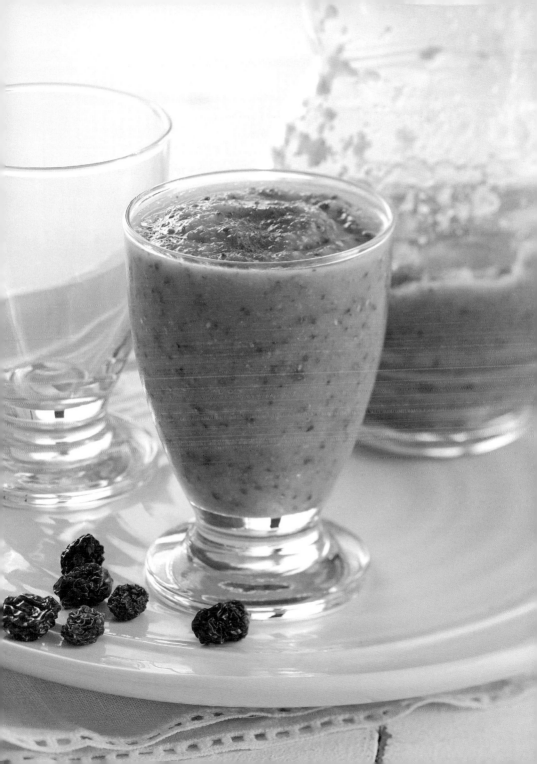

Velvety Banana Chia Pudding

This is a thick, rich, and subtly sweet pudding that is perfect for athletes and non-athletes alike. Protein-rich chia seeds combine with carbohydrate- and electrolyte-rich bananas to help you fuel and refuel. Enjoy a satiating ½-cup (75 g) serving (or more) pre- or post-workout or any time you need a quick, convenient, and nourishing meal or snack.

2   **cups (475 ml) unsweetened coconut milk**
4   **pitted dates**
2   **medium bananas**
½   **teaspoon pure vanilla extract**
⅓   **cup (66.5 g) chia seeds**
    Honey, to taste (optional)

Combine the coconut milk, dates, bananas, and vanilla extract in a high-speed blender and blend until smooth. Pour into a container with a tight-fitting lid (I like to use a mason jar or Pyrex storage dish), add the chia seeds, and shake. Alternatively, you can pour the liquid into a separate bowl and stir in the chia seeds to combine. Let the pudding rest for 30 minutes, shaking or stirring every 5 to 10 minutes, until thick.

Pour the pudding into serving bowls, drizzle with honey, and serve.

Yield: Serves 3 or 4

Power Muesli

Whole-grain oats form the base of this simple, whole food–based breakfast "cereal." It's packed with protein and healthy fats from three super seeds (chia, hemp, and sunflower) and boasts the energy-boosting power and sweet-tart flavor of vitamin B–rich goldenberries. Make a double or triple batch of this muesli and store in the freezer for a convenient, ready-to-eat breakfast or snack.

2	cups (160 g) rolled oats (see Note)
½	cup (75 g) dried currants
½	cup (60 g) dried goldenberries
¼	cup (30 g) hemp seeds
¼	cup (50 g) chia seeds
¼	cup (36 g) sunflower seeds
	Honey, to taste (optional)

Combine all of the ingredients in a large bowl. Store in an airtight container. This keeps best refrigerated or frozen.

For a cold muesli: In a serving bowl, combine ¼ cup (20 g) muesli with ¼ cup (60 ml) coconut milk (or other milk) per serving. Soak for 5 to 10 minutes or overnight, drizzle with honey to taste, and serve.

For a warm muesli: In a small saucepan, combine ¼ cup (20 g) muesli with ¼ cup (60 ml) coconut milk (or other milk) per serving. Bring to a boil, remove from the heat, and drizzle with honey to taste. Serve warm.

Yield: About 3½ cups (300 g)

Note: This recipe is gluten-free if you choose to use gluten-free rolled oats. Although traditional oats do not contain wheat, barley, or rye (all of which contain gluten), they may become contaminated with these gluten-containing grains during processing. For this reason, if you are following a gluten-free diet, consume only oats labeled "gluten-free."

Creamy Broccoli & Potato Soup

When I advise clients to avoid "white foods," I do not include potatoes (or cauliflower or parsnips, for that matter) on that list. Potatoes
are a nutrient-rich source of carbohydrates for energy, and together,
broccoli and potatoes are packed with vitamins and minerals. One
cup (71 g) of chopped broccoli boasts nearly 300 milligrams of potassium, while one medium potato contains nearly 900 milligrams
of potassium—meeting more than 20 percent of your estimated
daily need when combined. Enjoy this creamy soup, which uses chia
as a thickener (and to provide a small boost of protein and fat), alone
or topped with a sprinkle of shredded Cheddar cheese.

2   teaspoons extra-virgin olive oil
½   medium onion, chopped
4   cups (284 g) fresh broccoli florets
     (or thawed frozen)
1½   pounds (680 g) white potatoes,
     peeled and chopped into 1-inch
     (2.5 cm) chunks
4   cups (950 ml) vegetable broth
1   tablespoon (12.5 g) milled
     chia seeds
     Sea salt and freshly ground black
     pepper, to taste
     Shredded Cheddar cheese, for
     topping (optional)

In a large pot, heat the oil over medium heat. Add the onion and sauté until it softens, about 3 minutes. Add the broccoli florets, potatoes, and vegetable broth to the pot (the vegetables will just barely be covered by the broth) and bring to a boil. Reduce the heat, cover, and simmer, stirring occasionally, until the vegetables are soft, about 10 to 15 minutes.

Remove from the heat and stir in the milled chia seeds. Using an immersion blender, blend the soup until it becomes smooth and creamy. (If you do not have an immersion blender, let the soup cool, puree in small batches in a high-speed blender, and return to the pot.) Season with sea salt and black pepper. Ladle into serving bowls, top with a generous sprin-kle of shredded Cheddar cheese, and serve.

Yield: Serves 6 to 8

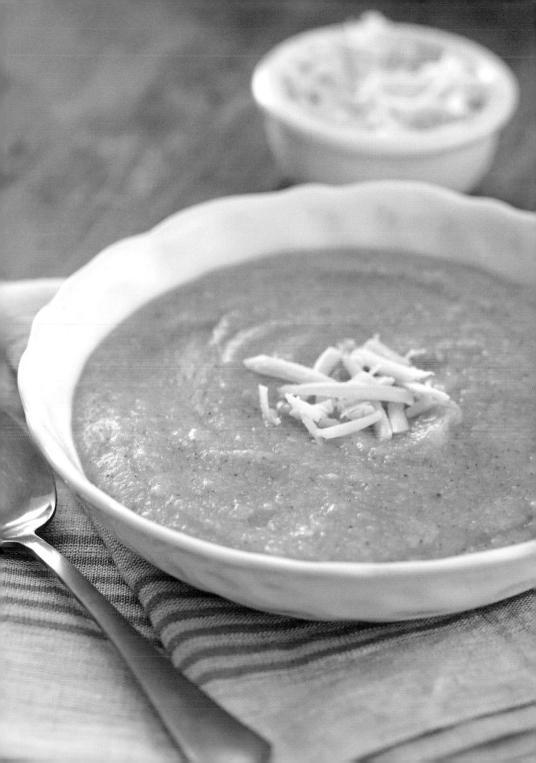

Lentil and Split Pea Salad with Sacha Inchi Seed Dressing

Lentils and split peas are packed with a combination of carbohydrates (about 40 grams per cup) and protein (about 18 grams per cup), making them an ideal food for sustained energy. And unlike dried beans, which need to be soaked overnight before they can be cooked, dried lentils can be rinsed and quickly prepared (no soaking needed)—ideal for the busy athlete in search of quick but nutrient-packed meals. Enjoy this hearty salad as a main meal or side dish. Sacha inchi seed oil is rich in omega-3 fatty acids, but if you are unable to find it at your local market, you can easily substitute with extra-virgin olive oil or hemp oil.

½   **cup (96 g) dried lentils**
½   **cup (113 g) dried split peas**
4   **cups (950 ml) water**
2   **carrots, peeled and finely chopped**
3   **tablespoons (37.5 g) chia seeds**
¼   **cup (60 ml) sacha inchi seed oil**
2   **tablespoons (28 ml) freshly squeezed lemon juice**
1   **tablespoon (4 g) chopped fresh parsley**
1   **tablespoon (10 g) chopped fresh shallots**
1   **teaspoon Dijon mustard**
1   **teaspoon honey**
    Sea salt and freshly ground black pepper, to taste

Rinse and drain the lentils and split peas. Place the lentils, split peas, and water in a medium saucepan. Bring to a boil, cover, reduce the heat, and simmer for about 30 minutes until the lentils and split peas are soft and tender (but not mushy). Remove from the heat and drain; rinse the lentils and sweet peas in cold water.

In a large bowl, stir together the lentils, split peas, carrots, and chia seeds.

In a small bowl, whisk together the oil, lemon juice, parsley, shallots, mustard, honey, sea salt, and black pepper. Drizzle the dressing over the salad and stir to combine. Season with additional sea salt and black pepper. Serve chilled.

Yield: Serves 4 to 6

Super Seed & Vegetable Dip

This zesty dip is a modified version of a seedless nut pâté I learned to make a few years ago in a raw food training session. In this recipe, I pack in the protein (and healthy fats) with a combination of sunflower, chia, and hemp seeds. In fact, this dip contains nearly 50 grams of protein, more than you would find in two chicken breasts. You will also get a big boost of antioxidant vitamin C with the addition of two whole red bell peppers, which each contain more than 75 milligrams of vitamin C. Serve this with fresh vegetable slices or crackers. You can also use it as a sandwich spread.

1   cup (145 g) raw sunflower seeds
¼   cup (50 g) chia seeds
2   tablespoons (15 g) hemp seeds
2   red bell peppers, seeded and chopped
2   stalks celery, chopped
2   scallions, chopped
¼ teaspoon sea salt, plus more to taste

Combine all of the ingredients in a food processor and process until moist and chunky. Transfer to an airtight container and refrigerate for at least 30 minutes before serving so that the flavors can develop and the dip can thicken. Serve chilled.

Yield: About 2½ cups

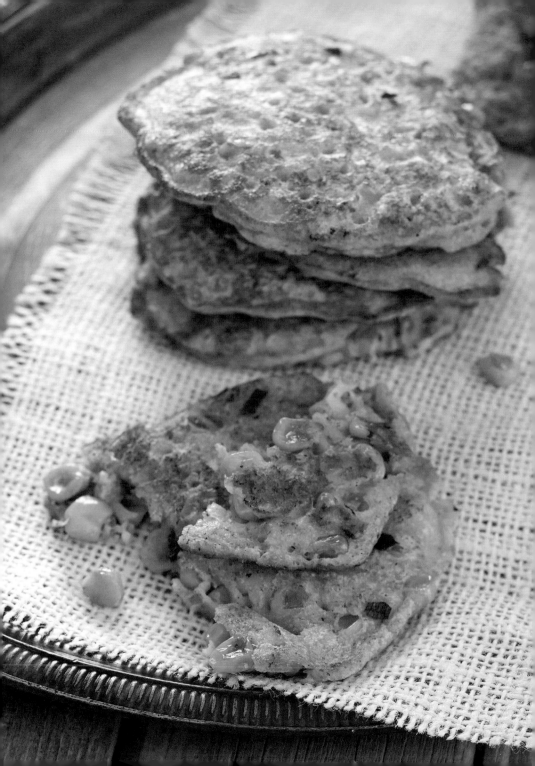

Chia Corn Cakes

A generous scoop of milled chia seeds is blended right into the batter of these hearty corn cakes, providing an extra boost of protein, fat, and fiber. Cayenne pepper offers both its flavor and inflammation-fighting power. Enjoy at mealtime as a main or side dish.

1 tablespoon (15 ml) canola oil, plus more for browning (preferably organic, expeller pressed)

2 cups (308 g) fresh corn kernels (or [328 g] thawed frozen)

3 scallions, thinly sliced

¾ cup (102 g) Bob's Red Mill all-purpose gluten-free baking flour

¼ cup (50 g) milled chia seeds

1 teaspoon sea salt

½ teaspoon baking powder

½ teaspoon Old Bay seasoning

Few generous pinches of cayenne pepper

1 cup (235 ml) whole or unsweetened coconut milk

1 large egg, beaten

Preheat the oven to 350°F (180°C, or gas mark 4). Heat the oil in a large skillet over medium-high heat. Add the corn and scallions and cook until soft and browned, stirring occasionally, 10 to 15 minutes.

In a large bowl, combine the flour, milled chia seeds, salt, baking powder, Old Bay seasoning, and cayenne pepper. Add the milk and beaten egg and mix until combined. Fold in the corn and scallions.

Wipe out the skillet, add a thin film of oil, and heat over medium to medium-high heat. Drop ¼ cup (60 ml) of batter onto the hot skillet per cake, being careful not to crowd the skillet, and cook until browned, 3 to 5 minutes per side. Continue until all of the batter has been used, adding more oil between batches as needed.

Transfer the corn cakes to a plate lined with paper towels to absorb any excess oil. Lay the cakes in a single layer on a baking sheet. Bake for 8 to 10 minutes. Serve warm.

Yield: 10 to 12 cakes

Cherry & Cashew Chia Clusters

This simple treat combines crunchy cashews and chia seeds with sweet bursts of inflammation-fighting cherries.

$\frac{1}{2}$ cup plus 2 tablespoons (200 g) honey

$\frac{1}{2}$ teaspoon pure vanilla extract
Pinch of sea salt

2 cups (280 g) raw cashews (1 cup whole, 1 cup roughly chopped)

$\frac{1}{2}$ cup (80 g) chopped unsweetened dried cherries

$\frac{1}{4}$ cup (50 g) chia seeds

Preheat the oven to 325°F (170°C, or gas mark 3). In a large bowl, whisk together the honey, vanilla, and sea salt. Stir in the whole and chopped cashews, cherries, and chia seeds and toss until the nuts are well coated. Transfer to a large baking sheet. Bake for about 15 minutes, stirring occasionally, until the nuts turn golden brown. Transfer to a surface lined with waxed paper and let cool completely. Break into small clusters and store in an airtight container or bag. The clusters keep best refrigerated or frozen.

Yield: 3½ to 4 cups (490 to 560 g)

Spicy Orange & Goji Berry Chia Fruit Leather

This convenient snack packs especially well for travel.

1 cup (235 ml) freshly squeezed orange juice

$\frac{1}{4}$ cup (23 g) dried goji berries

$\frac{1}{4}$ cup (50 g) chia seeds
Pinch of cayenne pepper

Combine the juice and berries in a blender until smooth. Transfer to a small bowl and stir in the chia seeds and cayenne pepper. Let rest for 30 minutes, stirring or shaking every 5 to 10 minutes, until a thick gel forms. Using a spatula, spread on a Teflex-lined dehydrator sheet in a very thin layer and shape the gel into a large square, which should cover more than three-quarters of the sheet. Dehydrate at 105°F (41°C) for about 3½ hours.

Remove the tray from the dehydrator and carefully flip the fruit leather over directly onto the mesh screen. Gently peel the Teflex sheet off. Place the tray back in the dehydrator and continue to dehydrate at 105°F (41°C) for an additional 30 minutes. The fruit leather is done when it is dry to the touch but still malleable and chewy

Transfer to a cutting board, and cut into twenty 1 x 6-inch (2.5 x 15 cm) strips. Store in an airtight container or bag.

Yield: 20 fruit leather strips

Crispy Almond Butter Energy Bars

These ooey-gooey, protein-packed crispy squares are a step up from the traditional marshmallow treats you may have enjoyed as a child. I like to use a combination of raw or roasted almond butter and semisweet chocolate chips, which contain more cacao and antioxidants than milk chocolate chips. My family enjoys bars that are thick and chunky, so I spread this mixture into a 9 x 13-inch (23 x 33 cm) baking dish. If you prefer a thinner bar, simply press the mixture onto a baking dish and cut into any size you choose.

6	cups (150 g) crispy brown rice cereal
1	cup (145 g) raw almonds, chopped
½	cup (87.5 g) chocolate chips
¼	cup (50 g) chia seeds
1	teaspoon ground cinnamon
1½	cups (390 g) almond butter
1½	cups (510 g) honey
1	teaspoon pure vanilla extract

In a medium bowl, stir together the cereal, almonds, chocolate chips, chia seeds, and cinnamon. In a large bowl, stir together the almond butter, honey, and vanilla extract. Add the dry ingredients to the wet—in 3 or 4 additions—mixing well after each addition. Continue to mix (using your fingertips, if necessary) to ensure the dry ingredients are thoroughly and evenly coated with the sticky almond butter and honey.

Spread the mixture into a 9 x 13-inch (23 x 33 cm) baking dish. Place a sheet of waxed paper on top and press down firmly over the entire surface with the palms of your hands. Refrigerate until firm, about 30 minutes.

Cut into 12 bars to serve. Keep refrigerated in an airtight container.

Yield: 12 bars

Chocolate & Maca Chia Chews

This the ultimate treat for chocolate and maca lovers! Three super-foods—raw cacao, raw maca, and chia seeds—unite in flavor and nutrition. Maca is an adaptogenic root that helps the body adapt to stress and naturally strengthens the systems of the body. And raw cacao powder is chock-full of antioxidants and compounds that may help boost mood and reduce stress. These energizing treats are perfect as an afternoon pick-me-up or for any time your body needs a revitalizing boost.

2   **cups (356 g) pitted dates**
½   **cup (43 g) shredded dried coconut**
2   **tablespoons (25 g) chia seeds**
1   **teaspoon pure vanilla extract**
2   **tablespoons (12 g) raw cacao powder**
2   **tablespoons plus 2 teaspoons (21 g) raw maca powder, divided**

Combine the dates, coconut, chia seeds, and vanilla extract in a food processor and pulse into a coarse and slightly sticky meal. The mixture should stick together when pressed with the fingertips. If it feels too dry, add one or two more dates and process. If it feels too sticky, add a tablespoon or two (5 to 10 g) of dried coconut and process. Add the cacao powder and 2 teaspoons of the maca to the to the mixture and process until combined into a slightly sticky "dough."

Place the remaining 2 tablespoons (16 g) maca powder in a small bowl. Roll the "dough" into teaspoon-size balls and dredge in the maca powder to coat. Store in an airtight container, or you can freeze for long-term storage.

Yield: 30 to 40 chews

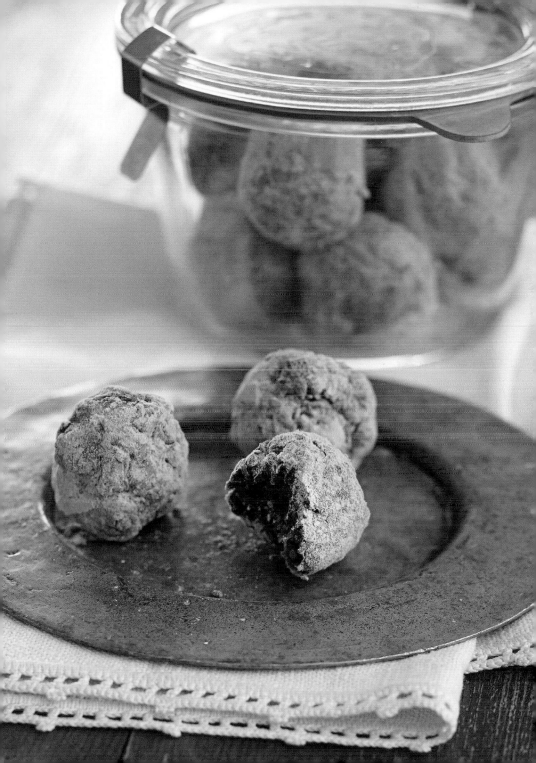

CHAPTER 3

The Healthy Gut: Using Chia to Support Digestion

Does your diet support your body's digestive system—or burden it? In today's world, many individuals are wreaking havoc on their digestion and overloading its ability to naturally detoxify by making poor food and lifestyle choices. Perhaps you consume too many processed foods and too few whole foods that are rich in the fiber, vitamins, minerals, and other nutrients your body needs to support digestion and detoxification. Or maybe you consume lots of conventionally raised meat and dairy products that contain growth hormones and antibiotics, the latter of which destroy both the "bad" and "good" health-promoting bacteria in your gut. Or perhaps you simply eat too much food in general, don't drink enough water, don't get enough sleep, or don't exercise regularly. You may even find yourself frequently stressed (did you know that your emotional state is also linked to digestion?) and suffering from constipation or diarrhea.

Indeed, a poor diet coupled with poor lifestyle choices can impair your digestion, but making better food choices can improve the health of your digestive tract and support your body's natural ability to detoxify. And when your gut is functioning better, you feel better. A healthy and optimally running digestive tract helps your body break down the food you eat, enhances nutrient absorption, boosts immunity (did you know that more than 70 percent of your immune system is located in and around your gut?), and supports daily detoxification by keeping waste matter moving through the intestines—and out of your body. So how can you foster a healthy digestive tract? Adding a little fiber to your diet—including my favorite go-to, fiber-rich chia seed—is a simple place to start. And in this chapter, I'll show you how.

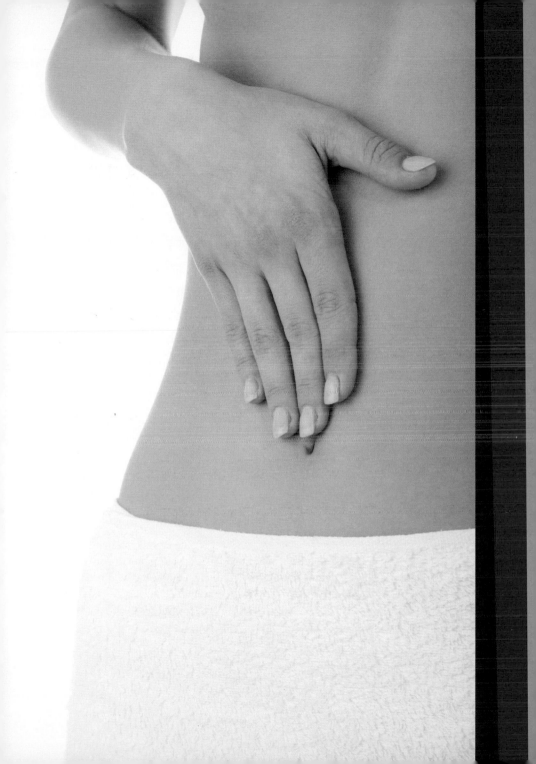

Fiber-Rich Chia Keeps the Bowels Moving

It's time to talk digestion—and elimination. As you may recall from Chapter 1, most Americans do not consume enough dietary fiber. In fact, the average person consumes only about 15 grams of dietary fiber each day—far below the recommended 25 to 35 daily grams for health and weight. And not surprisingly, the National Institutes of Health (NIH) reports that more than 4 million Americans suffer from frequent constipation (having a bowel movement fewer than three times per week). Being constipated can cause abdominal pain, nausea, and headaches. It can also lead to uncomfortable hemorrhoids, umbilical hernias, and diverticular disease (the presence of small pouches called diverticula in the colon). In addition, it is estimated that more than 725 million dollars are spent annually on laxative products. How did we get into this bind (pun intended)? And how can we get out?

Simply stated, a fiber-rich diet is key to regulating bowel function. And experts agree that adequate fiber intake—25 to 35 grams per day—is enough to prevent and relieve constipation and keep you regular. Fortunately, chia seeds are an incredibly easy, fiber-rich food to add to the diet to help regulate bowel movements and prevent constipation. Just 1 ounce (28.35 g) of seeds (2 to 2 ½ tablespoons), contains nearly 10 grams of dietary fiber—about 30 to 40 percent of your daily needs. And this relatively small amount of chia goes a long way in filling the gap between what most Americans are consuming (about 15 grams a day) and what they should be consuming (25 to 35 grams per day) for good health and digestion. In addition, chia seeds contain a nice balance of both soluble and insoluble fiber, the latter of which helps keep you "going" regularly.

In general, dietary fiber can be categorized into one of two types—soluble or insoluble—and plant foods typically contain a mixture of both. Soluble fiber dissolves in water and forms a gel-like substance in the intestines. It may help lower blood cholesterol and blood sugar levels in the body (you will learn more about this in the next chapter). Foods rich in soluble fiber include oats, beans, berries, and apples. By contrast, insoluble fiber does not dissolve in water and passes through the intestinal tract pretty much unchanged. It helps increase the weight and bulk of the stool to keep your bowels moving regularly. Foods rich in insoluble fiber include whole wheat, wheat bran, beans, most vegetables, and nuts and seeds—including chia seeds.

In fact, in a study published in 2010, researchers at the University of Arizona at Tucson found that approximately half of the fiber in chia seeds—about 40 to 60 percent—is in the form of elimination-friendly insoluble fiber. So if you find yourself frequently constipated and want to boost your fiber intake, chia seeds will be a great addition to the daily diet. You can also refer to Dietary Fiber Content of Various Plant Foods (page 20) to help guide you in selecting fiber-rich choices.

Fiber-Rich Foods May Help Ease Symptoms of IBS

Fiber-rich foods like chia seeds may also help promote regularity and reduce gas and bloating in those with irritable bowel syndrome (IBS). IBS is a disorder of the digestive tract that typically causes abdominal pain, bloating, distention, gas, and frequent constipation or diarrhea (usually both) with no clear physical cause. The NIH estimates that as few as 3 percent and as much as 20 percent of the population has IBS. Although the cause and treatment of IBS tends to be highly individual and complex, most experts agree that people with IBS should limit or avoid high-fat foods, dairy products, alcohol, caffeine, and some fiber-rich, gas-producing foods (like beans)—all of which may trigger symptoms. However, researchers have also found that gradually increasing fiber intake by 2 to 3 grams each day (the amount in 1½ teaspoons of chia seeds) may help ease symptoms like gas and bloating in some individuals with IBS. In addition, a fiber intake of 25 to 35 grams per day may also help lessen the constipation associated with it.

Naturally Gluten-Free, Fiber,- and Mineral-Rich Seed

Chia seeds also provide a wonderful, naturally gluten-free source of dietary fiber and minerals for those who have been diagnosed with celiac disease or gluten intolerance. Celiac disease is a digestive disease that affects the small intestine. Individuals with celiac disease cannot tolerate gluten (a protein found in wheat, barley, and rye), which causes damage to the lining of the small intestine when consumed. As a result, those with celiac disease must adhere to a strict gluten-free diet. By contrast, those with gluten intolerance or gluten sensitivity may present with similar symptoms as those with celiac disease, but consuming gluten-containing foods does not seem to damage the small intestine. Because fiber-rich whole grains are eliminated from the gluten-free diet, those with celiac disease or gluten intolerance may run the risk of too low fiber intake. Fortunately, fiber-rich chia seeds can help boost the fiber content of the diet for those who cannot consume whole grains—and in a small, nutrient-rich, simple-to-use package.

Additionally, because celiac disease causes damage to the lining of the small intestine, certain vitamins and minerals like calcium, iron, and B vitamins may not be well absorbed. An added benefit of chia seeds is that they are rich in a few of these important minerals. An ounce (28.35 g) of chia seeds contains over 2 milligrams of iron—about 10 to 25 percent of the average adult's needs. And ounce for ounce, chia seeds contain five times more calcium than milk, with nearly 200 milligrams per ounce. For individuals diagnosed with celiac disease, chia seeds provide a good source of these important minerals as the gut heals on a gluten-free diet.

DID YOU KNOW?

If you have diverticular disease (the presence of pouches in the co-lon) or diverticulitis (inflammation of those pouches), you may still be able to enjoy your favorite nuts and seeds—including chia seeds. In the past, physicians typically advised patients with diverticular disease to avoid all nuts and seeds, as it was thought that they could lodge into the pouches of the colon and cause pain and inflammation. But today, researchers believe that a high-fiber diet—even one that includes nuts and seeds—may reduce the risk of diverticular disease and flare-ups (or at least not trigger them) in those who have it. In fact, a low-fiber diet, chronic constipation, and straining during bowel movements are all thought to be causes of diverticular disease. If you have divertic-ular disease, ask your health care provider about experimenting with nutrient-dense, fiber-rich foods (like chia seeds) to determine which ones keep your digestive tract running smoothly and prevent—not cause—flare-ups.

Beyond Digestion:
Daily Detoxification with Fiber-Rich Chia

Eating fiber-rich foods like chia seeds helps keep your bowels moving and in doing so, supports your body's daily waste-removal efforts. As fiber moves through the intestines, it acts like a mop, soaking up and sweeping out anything your body does not need, like excess cholesterol, toxins, and waste. And this, I believe, is one of the most important and often overlooked aspects of detoxification.

Detox diets are becoming more and more popular, and nearly every week I see a new "cleanse" being advertised online or on the cover of a magazine. I have had clients embark on elimination diets (just because), master cleanses, 3-day (or more) juice cleanses, and combination juice and smoothie cleanses, all with what I believe is a misguided desire to detox their bodies (though I suspect that most of them simply want to lose weight). Although I believe periodic cleansing may offer benefits to both mind and body for some people, I also believe that real detoxification—and certainly the starting point for any short-term "cleanse" of your choosing—begins with your daily diet.

So what are you eating each day to support your body's ability to naturally detoxify and eliminate waste? I like to guide clients toward fiber, fluids, and nutrient-dense superfoods like chia. Consuming adequate fiber helps support your bowels and regular elimination; drinking enough water helps support the kidneys and their ability to remove waste through the urine; and eating more whole, organic foods (mainly vegetables, fruits, nuts, seeds, eggs, and wild fish) will give your body the nutrients it needs (like amino acids and vitamin C) to support your hard-working liver. The recipes in this chapter combine fiber- and protein-rich chia with a few of my favorite liver- and kidney-loving foods to support your body's daily natural detoxification processes—and help you look and feel your best.

SPOTLIGHT: PROBIOTICS AND PREBIOTICS

You may have heard that you can improve digestion by consuming more probiotic- and prebiotic-rich foods. Probiotics are the beneficial bacteria (like *Lactobacilli and Bifidobacteria*) found in fermented foods (like kombucha, kefir, miso, kimchi, and sauerkraut) and probiotic supplements. Prebiotics are non-digestible carbohydrates (like inulin and fructooligosaccharides [FOS]) that are fermented by and essentially "feed" the good bacteria in your gut. Foods rich in prebiotics include apples, berries, bananas, onions and garlic, leeks, Jerusalem artichokes, yacon root, and asparagus. Together, probiotics and the prebiotics that feed them may help improve digestion, enhance the absorption of nutrients in the small intestine, stimulate the immune system, and protect the body from invaders like "bad" bacteria, viruses, parasites, and other pathogens. (I like to think of the "good" bacteria as little soldiers that line the walls of the intestine to keep predators out.)

Although chia seeds are rich in fiber, as of this writing, I was unable to find any studies examining whether or not its fibers could be specifically classified as prebiotics (prebiotics must meet specific criteria to be classified as such). Certainly the fiber in chia seeds is beneficial to overall digestion, so in this chapter, I have combined the fiber-rich chia seed with some of my favorite prebiotic- and probiotic-rich foods to support digestive health.

Putting It into Practice

Chia seeds are one of the simplest fiber-rich foods that you can add to your diet to improve digestion and elimination. Here are a few simple diet (and lifestyle) tips to get you started on the path to a happy and healthy gut:

- *Boost your dietary fiber intake naturally—with chia seeds.* Add 1 ounce (28.35 g) of chia seeds (2 to 2½ tablespoons) to your daily diet to for an extra 10 grams of dietary fiber—the amount missing from most diets. You can sprinkle small amounts of chia seeds into your diet throughout the day as you build up to this intake (and perhaps discover that you require just a small amount to improve digestion). Try the Simple Morning Muesli (page 93) or Sweet Green Smoothie (page 92) for breakfast or the Apple, Pear, & Cinnamon Granola Bars (page 103) or Back-to-Basics Trail Mix (page 101) as a between-meal snack to help you meet your daily fiber needs.

- *Make friends with fermented foods.* Fermented foods contain the probiotics ("good" bacteria) that help support the digestive and immune systems. Miso, kombucha, kimchi, kefir, and sauerkraut are all good choices. You can also try the refreshing Super Berry Chia Bucha (page 89) as a hydrating and nourishing between-meal snack offering a boost of beneficial fiber (from chia seeds), probiotics (from kombucha), and antioxidants (from maqui berries). You can also check out some of the incredible recipes from *Fermented Foods for Health* (Fair Winds Press, 2013) by Deirdre Rawlings, Ph.D., N.D

- *Drink more water.* Staying hydrated helps prevent constipation and supports the kidneys and removal of waste products through the urine. Strive for at least 1 to 2 liters (1 to 2 quarts) of pure water each day—especially if you are starting to increase your fiber intake. Remember that increasing your fiber intake too rapidly (too much, too soon) without also increasing your fluid intake can cause abdominal pain, bloating, and constipation. So be sure to drink plenty of fluids as you gradually increase your fiber intake with chia seeds and other fiber-rich foods.

- *Choose organic when available and your budget allows.* According to the United States Department of Agriculture, organic crops are, by definition, produced without synthetic fertilizers, prohibited pesticides, irradiation, genetically modified organisms, and, yes—sewage sludge. Organic animal products are produced without the use of hormones or antibiotics and fed 100 percent organic feed. In essence, choosing organic food helps reduce your toxic load from the amount of pesticides, hormones, and antibiotics your body would otherwise be exposed to at each meal. And when you choose more organic whole foods (that grow in the ground or on a tree) and fewer processed foods (that come in a bag or box), you will help supply your body with the synergistic blend of nutrients it needs to support the important work of the liver, intestines, and kidneys.

- *Eat mindfully.* Chewing begins the process of digestion. Eating slowly and chewing thoroughly aids digestion. So slow down and savor each meal and snack.

- *Move more.* Building time into your weekly schedule for exercise—as simple as a brisk walk a few times a week—helps keep the bowels moving and may prevent constipation and ease the symptoms of irritable bowel syndrome. For those who enjoy more intense exercise—like running or hot yoga—sweating also aids the body in detoxification. So go ahead and sweat those toxins out!

- *Just say "om."* Stress can wreak havoc on your digestion, and indeed, experts recognize the connection between your brain and your gut. Reducing stress through deep breathing, visualization, or meditation may also help improve digestion.

SEE YOUR DOCTOR

There are several digestive disorders whose prevention and treatment is far more complex than the simple addition of a little fiber or water to your diet (and far too complex to be addressed in this chapter alone). Like many dietitians, I have typically seen patients with digestive issues after they have been diagnosed by or while under the care of their gastroenterologist. I may have helped guide them through an elimination diet (eliminating suspect foods from the diet for a short period of time followed by a period of reintroduction to see how the body responds to the suspect foods) to aid their doctor in diagnosis, or I might have provided dietary guidance based on their current diagnosis. However, if a client came to me with ongoing or acute digestive issues that have not yet been evaluated, I always recommended that they seek out the advice of their physician before making drastic changes to the diet or taking supplements—and I recommend you do the same.

Being evaluated by a specialist can help rule out more serious medical conditions like celiac disease or ovarian cancer, the latter of which may also cause abdominal pain, distention, and bloating. And it can also help determine the cause and course of treatment, which almost always includes dietary changes. In addition, making drastic changes to your diet before consulting with a specialist may cause symptoms to worsen or skew the results of certain diagnostic tests (for example, if you suspect you have celiac disease, you should not eliminate gluten from the diet before undergoing diagnostic testing, as celiac disease may not be picked up). Bottom line: If you are suffering from ongoing or acute abdominal or digestive issues, see your health care provider before making changes to your diet.

Chia-Inspired Recipes for a Healthy Gut

Lemony Chia Fresca

This traditional chia fresca has a citrusy and subtly sweet flavor. I often make a double or triple batch of this incredibly refreshing and simple-to-prepare beverage to have on hand, especially during the hot summer months, when I am craving a lemonade-style drink— but with extra fiber and without all the sugar of traditional lemonades.

2   cups (475 ml) water
3   tablespoons (45 ml) freshly squeezed lemon juice
2   teaspoons chia seeds
1   tablespoon (20 g) pure maple syrup

Combine the water, lemon juice, chia seeds, and maple syrup in a jar with a tight-fitting lid (I like to use a mason jar) and shake to combine. Let stand for about 10 minutes, shaking once or twice.

Serve chilled. Refrigerate any unused portion in an airtight container for 2 to 3 days.

Yield: Serves 1 to 2

Apple & Fennel Chia Elixir

This sweet beverage is an elixir for a troubled tummy. Sweet apples and the licorice-like flavor and bloat-busting power of fennel combine nicely with cinnamon, a super spice that not only helps balance blood sugars, but may also help ease nausea. If you need to be gentle to your digestive tract, reduce the fiber by using fewer chia seeds (a teaspoon or less).

3   medium apples
2   medium fennel bulbs
2   teaspoons chia seeds
    Pinch of ground cinnamon

Push the apples and fennel bulbs through a juicer (they should yield 1½ to 2 cups [355 to 475 ml] of juice). Stir in the chia seeds and let stand for about 10 minutes, stirring once or twice.

Pour into 1 or 2 glasses, sprinkle with cinnamon, and serve chilled. Refrigerate any unused portion in an airtight container for 2 to 3 days.

Yield: Serves 1 to 2

Super Berry Chia Bucha

This fizzy and fruity beverage combines chart-topping levels of antioxidants from dried maqui berry powder, the fiber-rich muscle of chia seeds, and the probiotic power of kombucha, a fermented tea beverage that is good for your gut.

2   cups (475 ml) plain kombucha
2   teaspoons maqui berry powder
1   teaspoon freshly squeezed lime juice
2   teaspoons chia seeds
    Honey, to taste (optional)

Combine the kombucha, maqui berry powder, lime juice, chia seeds, and honey in a large glass jar with a tight-fitting lid (I like to use a mason jar) and stir or very gently shake to combine (note that kombucha should not be vigorously shaken, as it is carbonated). Let stand for about 10 minutes, stirring or gently shaking once or twice.

Serve chilled. Refrigerate any unused portion in an airtight container for 2 to 3 days.

Yield: Serves 1 to 2

Sparkling Cranberry & Clementine Chia Fresca

The tart cranberry is a superstar when it comes to promoting good health, including gut health. These super berries contain heart-healthy, cancer-fighting antioxidants and phytochemicals, and they are uniquely rich in infection-fighting compounds that help keep bacteria from sticking to the walls of the bladder and stomach, including the stomach ulcer–promoting bacteria, *Helicobacter pylori*. The bitter flavor of freshly pressed cranberries is a perfect match for sweet clementines in this sparkling drink—no added sugar needed.

2   **cups (200 g) fresh cranberries (or thawed frozen)**
10 **clementines, peeled**
6   **cups (1.4 L) sparkling water, chilled**
2   **tablespoons (25 g) chia seeds**

Push the cranberries and clementines through a juicer (they should yield about 2 cups [475 ml] of juice). Transfer the juice to a large pitcher, add the sparkling water, and stir in the chia seeds. Let stand for about 10 minutes, stirring once or twice.

Pour into glasses and serve chilled. Refrigerate any unused portion in an airtight container for 2 to 3 days.

Yield: Serves 6 to 8

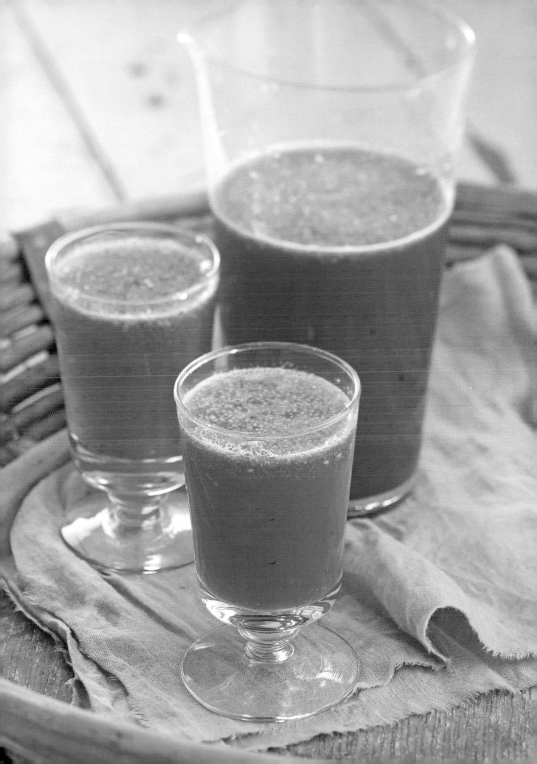

Sweet Green Smoothie

Green plant foods are highly alkalizing and detoxifying. And leafy greens—like the mild-tasting spinach that is used in this recipe—are also a rich source of important vitamins and minerals like vitamin A, vitamin K, folate, and iron. And when greens are blended into a smoothie like this one, your body not only soaks up their beneficial nutrients but also gets a gentle, "pre-digested" boost of its dietary fiber (more than 10 grams in this recipe), thanks to the blender's ability to "chew" your food for you.

1½ **cups (355 ml) water**
1 **cup (187 g) frozen pineapple chunks**
1 **cup (30 g) tightly packed spinach**
2 **stalks celery, chopped**
1 **cucumber, sliced (peeled if not organic)**
Juice of 1 lemon
3 **tablespoons (12 g) fresh parsley**
1 **tablespoon (12.5 g) chia seeds**

Combine all of the ingredients in a high-speed blender and blend until smooth.

Yield: Serves 1 to 2

Simple Morning Muesli

Enjoy this simple-to-make breakfast that combines the fiber-rich power of whole-grain rolled oats, dried fruit, and chia. I like to make a double or triple batch of this recipe and store it in the refrigerator or freezer so that I always have a healthy breakfast cereal on hand.

2   cups (160 g) rolled oats (see Note)
½   cup (50 g) raw walnuts, chopped
½   cup (75 g) golden raisins
½   cup (65 g) dried apricots, chopped
¼   cup (50 g) chia seeds
¼   cup (28 g) wheat germ (optional; see Note)
    Honey, to taste (optional)

Combine all of the ingredients in a large bowl. Store in an airtight container. This keeps best refrigerated or frozen.

For a cold muesli: In a serving bowl, combine ¼ cup (20 g) muesli with ¼ cup (60 ml) coconut milk (or other nondairy milk) per serving. Soak for 5 to 10 minutes or overnight, drizzle with honey to taste, and serve.

For a warm muesli: In a small saucepan, combine ¼ cup (20 g) muesli with ¼ cup (60 ml) coconut milk per serving. Bring to a boil, remove from the heat, and drizzle with honey to taste. Serve warm.

Yield: 3½ cups (300 g)

Note: This recipe is gluten-free if you omit the wheat germ and use gluten-free rolled oats. Although traditional oats do not contain wheat, barley, or rye (all of which contain gluten), they may become contaminated with these gluten-containing grains during processing. For this reason, if you are following a gluten-free diet, consume only oats labeled "gluten-free."

Carrot & Currant Salad with Sea Buckthorn Berry Dressing

This mildly sweet salad is tossed with a zesty dressing made from the juice of the tart sea buckthorn berry. Sometimes referred to as "nature's multivitamin," sea buckthorn berries are one of the richest known sources of vitamin C and contain a beneficial blend of fatty acids that may help prevent constipation and ulcers and heal the lining of the digestive tract. Enjoy this nourishing salad alone or added to your favorite leafy green salad.

1½ **cups (225 g) dried currants**

4 **cups (440 g) shredded carrots**

2 **tablespoons (25 g) chia seeds**

3 **tablespoons (45 ml) extra-virgin olive oil**

2 **tablespoons (30 ml) pure sea buckthorn berry juice**

2 **teaspoons agave syrup**

Pinch of sea salt

Soak the currants in warm water to rehydrate for about 15 minutes. Drain well.

In a bowl, combine the currants, carrots, and chia seeds and toss to combine. In a small bowl, whisk together the olive oil, sea buckthorn berry juice, agave syrup, and sea salt. Drizzle the dressing over the salad, toss, and serve or refrigerate until ready to serve.

Yield: Serves 4 to 6

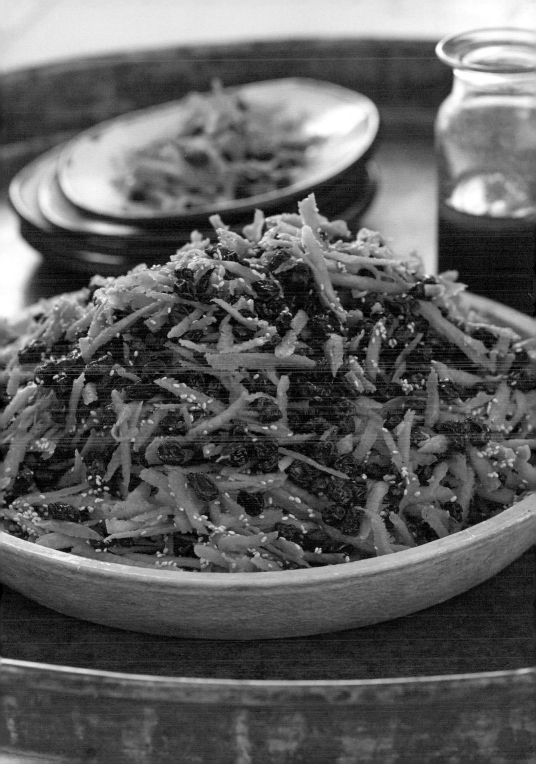

Endive Boats with Apple Salsa

This apple salsa is a crunchy and flavorful dish that combines the fiber-rich power of chopped figs, apples, and chia seeds. Naturally sweet figs are packed with calcium (nearly 250 milligrams of calcium per cup [150 g]) and boast nearly 15 grams of dietary fiber per cup [150 g]. And gut-friendly, prebiotic-rich apples are a great fruit for digestive health; their peels boast more than a dozen different cancer-fighting compounds. Enjoy this salsa on endive leaves, alone as a snack, or added to your favorite leafy green salad.

3   **apples, cored and finely chopped**

10   **dried figs (Calimyrna or Black Mission), finely chopped**

2 or 3 **small shallots, diced**

2   **teaspoons chia seeds**

1   **tablespoon (15 ml) freshly squeezed lemon juice**

1   **teaspoon extra-virgin olive oil**

1   **teaspoon honey**

     Pinch of sea salt

2   **heads red or white Belgian endive**

Place the apples, figs, shallots, chia seeds, lemon juice, olive oil, honey, and salt in a large bowl and stir together until well combined. Trim the ends off of the endive and place 1 heaping tablespoon (15 g) of apple salsa onto each leaf. Keep refrigerated until ready to serve. Serve chilled.

Yield: About 36 filled leaves

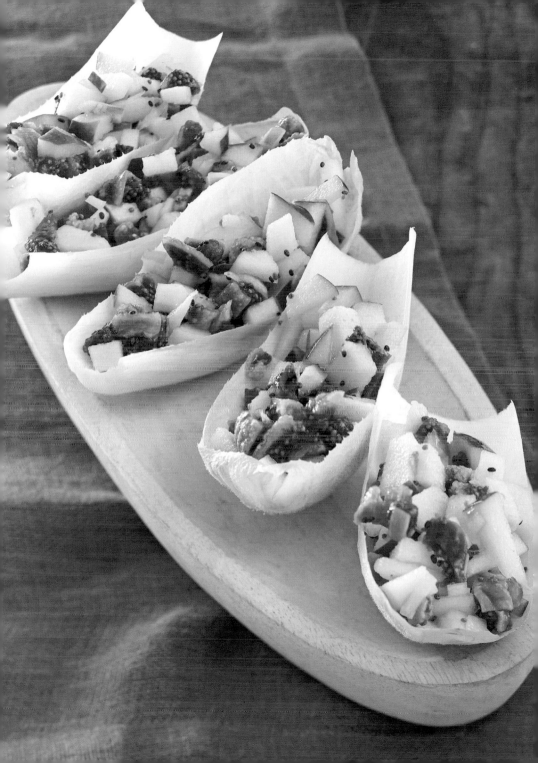

Asparagus & Leek Soup with Swirled Cashew Cream

Asparagus and leeks are both rich in prebiotics, which help feed the "good" bacteria in the gut to support digestion, enhanced nutrient absorption, and immunity. And asparagus is a rich source of glutathione, a compound found in Brussels sprouts and kale that helps detoxify certain carcinogens. Enjoy this soup on a chilly spring day—when asparagus and leeks are in season—topped with a thick cashew cream, which adds to the richness of the soup.

2	tablespoons (28 ml) extra-virgin olive oil
3	large leeks, sliced
2	bunches asparagus (about 1½ pounds, or 680 g), trimmed and cut into 1-inch (2.5 cm) pieces
4	cups (950 ml) vegetable broth
½	cup (70 g) raw cashews, soaked in water 6 to 8 hours
½	cup (120 ml) water
2	tablespoons (25 g) milled chia seeds
¼	teaspoon ground nutmeg
	Sea salt and freshly ground black pepper, to taste

Heat the oil in a large pot over medium heat. Add the sliced leeks and sauté until soft, about 5 minutes. Add the asparagus and vegetable broth and bring to a boil. Reduce the heat, cover, and simmer, stirring occasionally, until the asparagus has softened, 10 to 15 minutes.

While the soup is simmering, drain and rinse the cashews and place them in a high-speed blender with the water. Blend on high speed until smooth and creamy. Set aside.

Remove the soup from the heat and stir in the milled chia seeds. Blend with an immersion blender until smooth and creamy. (If you do not have an immersion blender, let the soup cool, puree in small batches in a high-speed blender, and return to the pot.) Season with sea salt and black pepper.

Stir the cashew cream into the soup, or ladle the soup into serving bowls and swirl each bowl with 1 to 2 teaspoons of cashew cream. Serve warm.

Yield: Serves 6 to 8

Celeriac & Potato Mash

I get celeriac (celery root) from my CSA every fall and winter, and I use it to make soups and this celeriac and potato mash—with a sprinkle of chia seeds for added fiber. Like potatoes, celeriac is a rich source of potassium, and it may confer some of the same benefits to digestion as celery itself, including easing gastritis, healing the lining of the stomach, and decreasing the risk of ulcers.

1   pound (455 g) celeriac, peeled and chopped into 1- to 2-inch (2.5 to 5 cm) cubes

1   pound (455 g) white potatoes, peeled and chopped into 1- to 2-inch (2.5 to 5 cm) cubes

3   tablespoons (45 ml) extra-virgin olive oil

1   tablespoon (12.5 g) chia seeds
    Sea salt and freshly ground black pepper, to taste

Place the celeriac in a large pot of water and bring to a boil. Boil the celeriac for 2 to 3 minutes. Add the potatoes and continue boiling for an additional 10 to 12 minutes until the vegetables are soft. Drain well.

Push the celeriac and potatoes through a ricer and into a large bowl. Stir in the olive oil and chia seeds. Season with sea salt and black pepper and serve warm.

Yield: Serves Serves 4 to 6

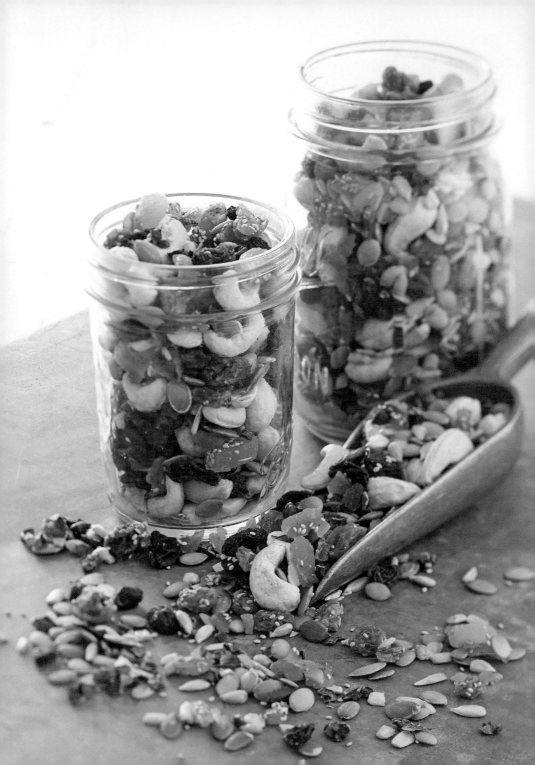

Back-to-Basics Trail Mix

Trail mix is a simple, satiating, protein- and fiber-rich between-meal snack. The best way to incorporate chia seeds into a trail mix is to toss them with sticky fruits, as they will cling to the fruits rather than settling to the bottom of the bag. Make a batch (or two or three) of this trail mix and store in a jar in your pantry (or refrigerator or freezer) for any time you crave a sweet and crunchy snack with a boost of fiber.

½ cup (75 g) raisins

½ cup (75 g) golden raisins

½ cup (65 g) dried apricots, finely chopped

1 tablespoon (12.5 g) chia seeds

1 cup (140 g) raw cashews

½ cup (32 g) raw pumpkin seeds

¼ cup (36 g) raw sunflower seeds

¼ cup (32 g) raw cacao nibs

In a large bowl, combine the dried fruits and chia seeds. Use your fingers to combine and gently press the chia seeds onto the dried fruit pieces. Mix in the remaining ingredients and store in an airtight container. This keeps best refrigerated or frozen.

Yield: About 3½ cups (525 g)

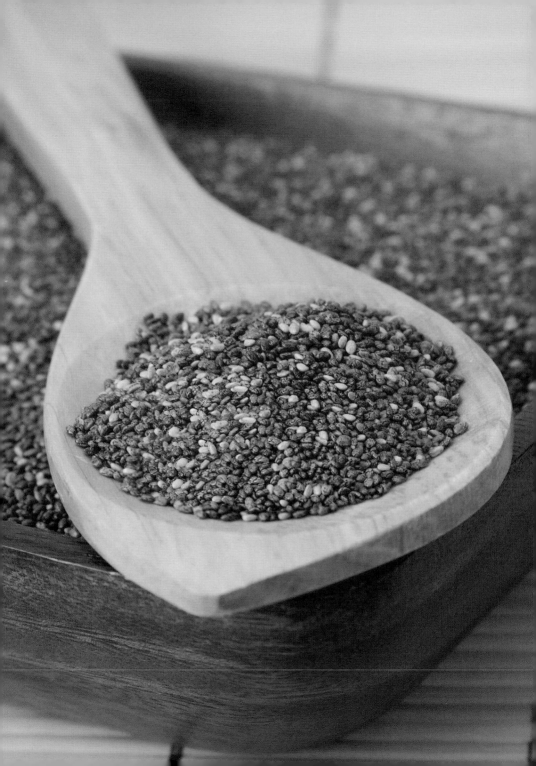

Apple, Pear & Cinnamon Granola Bars

This whole-food granola bar is a perfect fiber-rich fall snack. The natural sweetness of dehydrated, prebiotic-rich apples and pears combined with inflammation-fighting and nausea-quelling cinnamon and healthful fats and protein from a combination of four super seeds results in a chewy, fiber-rich bar. Enjoy at home or on the go.

2	apples, cored and chopped
2	pears, cored and chopped
2	teaspoons freshly squeezed lemon juice
¼	cup (50 g) chia seeds
¼	cup (42 g) whole flaxseeds
¼	cup (16 g) raw pumpkin seeds
¼	cup (36 g) raw sunflower seeds
1	teaspoon ground cinnamon
½	teaspoon pure vanilla extract
	Pinch of sea salt

Place the apples, pears, and lemon juice in a food processer and process into a moist, thick, and chunky mixture. Transfer the fruit to a large bowl and stir in the seeds, cinnamon, vanilla extract, and sea salt.

Using a spatula, spread the "dough" onto a Teflex-lined dehydrator sheet. Use the edge of the spatula to shape it into an approximately 10-inch (25 cm) square that's ½ inch (1 cm) thick. Dehydrate at 105°F (41°C) for about 24 hours until dry but still soft.

Remove the tray from the dehydrator and carefully flip the granola over onto a cutting board. Gently peel the Teflex sheet off of the granola, and cut into eight 2½ x 5-inch (6 x 13 cm) bars. Place the individual bars on the mesh screen and continue to dehydrate at 105°F (41°C) for an additional 10 to 12 hours. The granola bars are done when they are firm, dry, and slightly chewy. Store in an airtight container.

Yield: 8 bars

CHAPTER 4

Prime Health: Chia for a Strong Heart and Better Blood Sugars

The tiny chia seed is a powerhouse of disease-fighting nutrients, including inflammation-quelling omega-3 fatty acids, heart-healthy fiber, and cell-protecting antioxidants. And, of course, chia's rich blend of protein, fat, fiber, and carbohydrates helps keep your blood sugars—and your energy levels—steady. Not surprisingly, researchers are finding that chia seeds—and the nutrients in them—may help improve blood sugars, prevent the growth and spreading of certain types of cancer cells, and lower some of the risk factors associated with heart disease, like high cholesterol and blood pressure levels. In this chapter, you will learn about the heart-strong and blood sugar–balancing effects of chia seeds and how to add this super seed to your diet for its health-promoting power.

Omega-3 Alternative to Fish Oil

Chia seeds are an excellent source of the plant-based omega-3 fatty acid alpha-linolenic acid (ALA). Omega-3 fatty acids are heart-healthy polyunsaturated fats that include ALA, which is found only in plant foods, and DHA (docosahexaenoic acid) and EPA (eicosapentaenoic acid), which are most commonly found in oily cold-water fish like salmon and sardines. As a group, omega-3 fatty acids may help reduce inflammation, boost brain development and health, ease the pain and inflammation associated with arthritis, and lower the risk of heart disease. Although there is plenty of strong scientific evidence supporting the health benefits of EPA and DHA specifically, researchers are finding that ALA (which is converted to EPA and DHA in the body) may offer similar benefits to health, including heart health. Diets rich in ALA may help lower blood pressure and cholesterol levels and reduce the overall risk of heart disease and sudden death from heart attack. In fact, researchers have found that as intakes of ALA-rich foods rise, rates of death from heart disease and heart attacks seem to decline. For this reason, ALA-rich foods like chia seeds are a great option for boosting omega-3 fatty acid intake and heart health—especially for those who do not consume DHA- and EPA-rich fish or fish oil supplements.

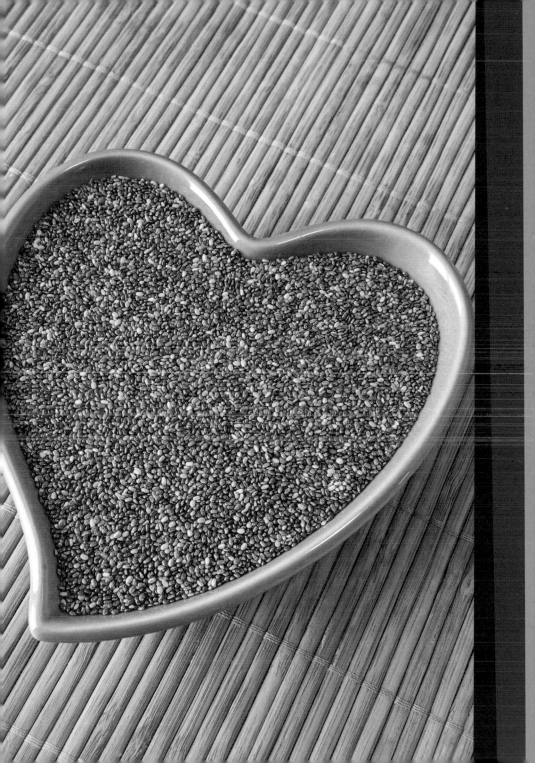

Indeed, chia seeds are reported to be one of the richest plant sources of ALA (with even more ALA than an equivalent serving of flaxseeds), although other good sources include flaxseeds, sacha inchi seeds, and walnuts. An ounce (about 2 to 2½ tablespoons, or 28.35 grams) of chia seeds contains almost 9 grams of total fat, and more than 75 percent of that fat is in the form of polyunsaturated fatty acids, including ALA. When fed to animals, ALA-rich chia seeds have been found to increase the omega-3 fatty acid content of their eggs, meat, and milk. And in human studies, researchers have found that when chia seeds are added to the diet, subjects' plasma levels of ALA and EPA tend to rise. In a small study published in 2012 in *Plant Foods in Human Nutrition*, researchers found that when

SPOTLIGHT: HEART DISEASE

Heart disease (sometimes called cardiovascular disease) broadly describes a number of conditions of the heart and blood vessels, including angina (chest pain), heart failure, arrhythmias (irregular heartbeat), and coronary artery disease, the latter of which is the most common type of heart disease, according to the Centers for Disease Control and Prevention (CDC). Coronary artery disease occurs when the arteries become narrow and hard due to the buildup of fatty plaques—a condition called atherosclerosis. It can cause reduced blood flow, lack of oxygen to the heart, and eventually lead to heart attack and death. Indeed, heart disease continues to be the leading killer of both men and women in the United States; the CDC estimates that about 600,000 people die from heart disease each year.

In addition to a family history of heart disease, other risk factors include high blood pressure, high cholesterol levels, inflammation of the blood vessels, obesity, and diabetes. Controllable factors like cigarette smoking, excessive alcohol consumption, lack of physical activity, stress, and a poor diet can also increase your risk of heart disease. In this chapter, I provide a few simple dietary recommendations—including the use of chia seeds—to support heart health.

10 postmenopausal women consumed 25 grams (about 2 tablespoons) of ground chia seeds daily for 7 weeks, their levels of ALA and EPA increased by 138 percent and 30 percent, respectively. And in a study published in 2012, rats fed chia oil for 3 weeks had increased plasma and tissue levels of omega-3 fatty acids—along with a decreased omega-6 to omega-3 fatty acid ratio. (See the "Did You Know?" text box below for more information on the importance of omega-6 to omega-3 ratios.) These results were similar to an earlier 2007 study, which found that rats fed chia (including whole chia seeds, ground chia seeds, and chia oil) all had significantly increased plasma levels of ALA, EPA, and DHA compared to the chia-free control diet—and an improved ratio of omega-6 to omega-3 fatty acids.

 DID YOU KNOW?

Both omega-6 and omega-3 fatty acids are important for health, and experts recommend consuming them in a 1:1 ratio for optimal health. Unfortunately, most Americans consume them in a 10:1 ratio—taking in too many omega-6 fatty acids in the form of vegetable oils from processed foods. And consuming too many omega-6 fats can cause inflammation, which may set the stage for chronic diseases like heart disease.

To help balance your intake of omega-6 and omega-3 fatty acids, I recommend reducing your intake of processed foods (like packaged crackers, chips, and cookies) and boosting your intake of omega-3-rich whole foods. You can include two or three weekly servings of DHA- and EPA-rich, fatty cold-water fish (like wild salmon and sardines) or seaweed, as well as a daily serving or two of ALA-rich nuts and seeds like chia seeds, flaxseeds, sacha inchi seeds, and walnuts. Chia seeds are an especially good and simple-to-add source of omega-3 fats in the diets of those who do not consume fish or fish oils.

Chia Seeds May Help Improve Blood Lipids and Blood Sugars

Studies have found that adding chia seeds to the diets of obese or insulin-resistant rats helps reduce elevated blood lipids (like cholesterol and triglycerides), improve insulin resistance and blood sugar control, and reduce visceral fat (the fat around the organs). In a 2007 study, researchers at the University of Arizona at Tucson found that rats whose diets consisted of whole chia seeds experienced significant decreases in triglycerides, while those consuming ground chia seeds had significant increases in HDL ("good") cholesterol levels. And in a more recent 2012 study, researchers found that rats whose high-fat, high-carbohydrate diets were supplemented with 5 percent chia seeds over an 8-week period had reduced inflammation in the heart and liver, decreased abdominal and liver fat, and improved insulin sensitivity and glucose tolerance compared to the control group. Similar results have been seen in humans.

In a study published in 2007 in *Diabetes Care*, researchers looked at the effects of a chia-enriched diet in 20 subjects with type 2 diabetes. For 12 weeks, subjects consumed 37 grams of chia (nearly 3 tablespoons) or wheat bran daily. Researchers found that the plasma levels of ALA and EPA doubled in subjects who consumed chia, while decreases were seen in certain markers for inflammation and proteins involved in blood clotting. Additionally, those consuming a chia-enriched diet also had a lower systolic blood pressure (the top number in a blood pressure reading that measures the force of blood in the arteries as the heart beats). High systolic blood pressure, if not treated, can lead to heart attack, stroke, or kidney damage. Adding chia to the diet also helped improve blood sugar control, evident by the significant decreases seen in subjects' hemoglobin A1C, a measure of long-term blood sugar control.

SPOTLIGHT: DIABETES

Diabetes is a metabolic disorder in which blood sugar levels are elevated due to the inability of the pancreas to produce sufficient insulin (a hormone that helps transport blood sugars to the cells of the body) or the inability of the body's cells to respond to insulin that is produced. It is classified as one of two types: type 1 diabetes (formerly called insulin-dependent diabetes) or type 2 diabetes (formerly called noninsulin-dependent diabetes). Type 1 diabetes is an autoimmune disease in which the body "attacks" the pancreas, causing it to produce little or no insulin. Type 2 diabetes is usually caused by insulin resistance (the inability of the body to use the insulin the pancreas produces) and is most commonly associated with a family history of diabetes, previous history of gestational diabetes (elevated blood sugars during pregnancy), obesity, older age, and lack of physical activity.

According to the National Institutes of Health, an estimated 23.6 million Americans have diabetes—that's nearly 8 percent of the population. And of those numbers, 90 to 95 percent have been diagnosed with type 2 diabetes. Symptoms and complications of diabetes may include increased thirst and urination, weight loss, hunger, fatigue, nerve damage, vision problems, and kidney disease. In some cases, undiagnosed or untreated diabetes can lead to coma and death. In most cases, diabetes, particularly type 2 diabetes, can be prevented with diet and lifestyle modifications and treated with a combination of diet and lifestyle measures along with medication. If you have been diagnosed with diabetes, see a registered dietitian or certified diabetes educator for advice—and ask about using chia seeds and other blood sugar–friendly foods to support its management.

In a more recent study published in 2012 in the *Journal of Nutrition*, researchers from Mexico looked at the effects of a reduced-calorie diet—with and without the addition of a "functional food"-based beverage that consisted of soy protein, nopal (also known as prickly pear), 4 grams of chia seeds, and oats—on the blood sugars and lipids of 67 subjects with metabolic syndrome (a group of risk factors that raises your risk of heart disease, diabetes, and stroke). After 2 months, both groups lost weight and reduced both their body mass index and waist circumference on their reduced-calorie diets. However, those consuming the beverage also had decreases in triglycerides, blood sugars, and C-reactive protein (a marker for inflammation), which researchers attributed to the combination of antioxidants, fiber, and fatty acids in these functional foods—including the added 4 grams of chia seeds.

Beyond Weight: Fiber-Rich Diets Reduce the Risk of Heart Disease

As you know, chia seeds are a rich source of dietary fiber that may help improve blood sugars, support heart health, and lower the risk of certain cancers. As you learned in the previous chapter, chia seeds contain both insoluble fiber (which is especially good for digestion and elimination) and heart-healthy soluble fiber. In general, when it comes to dietary fiber and health, studies have shown that the more fiber and whole grains you consume (see Spotlight: Whole Grains on page 19 for more information), the more likely you are to weigh less and the less likely you are to have heart disease, cancer, or type 2 diabetes. In fact, researchers have found that reducing fat in the diet (to less than 30 percent of calories from all fat and less than 10 percent of calories from saturated fat) and increasing dietary fiber intake from whole foods (about 6 servings per day from a combination of vegetables, fruits, and whole grains) may reduce your risk of heart disease and some types of cancer. As with weight maintenance, 25 to 35 grams of fiber per day is recommended for health. And some studies have found that by adding just 10 grams of fiber to your diet each day—the amount most Americans are missing from their daily diets—you could reduce the risk of dying from heart disease by as much as 35 percent. With nearly 10 grams of fiber per ounce, fiber-rich chia seeds are a simple way to boost your fiber intake and reap beneficial health effects.

Fiber-Rich Chia Seeds Help Improve Blood Sugars and Blood Lipids

As discussed in Chapter 1, because fiber-rich foods like chia are filling, they may help curb hunger and reduce the amount of food you eat each day, which may help you lose weight or maintain a healthy weight. This is important because simply being overweight or obese is a risk factor for chronic diseases like heart disease and diabetes. Fiber also helps slow digestion and the release of blood sugars into the bloodstream, which translates into more stable blood sugars for you. As you may recall from Chapter 1, a small study published in 2010 in the *European Journal of Clinical Nutrition* found that subjects who consumed chia-enriched breads (in amounts that included up to a maximum of 2 tablespoons [25 g] of ground chia) reported reduced appetites within 2 hours of consuming the bread—and had a dose-dependent reduction in blood sugars after eating the bread (meaning that the more chia baked into the bread, the lower their blood sugars after consuming it). Indeed, researchers found that for each gram (about ¼ teaspoon) of chia baked into the bread, post-meal blood sugars dropped 2 percent compared to the control group.

Dietary fiber—especially soluble fiber—also helps stimulate the release of bile (a digestive fluid that helps break down fats), which may help reduce both total and LDL ("bad") cholesterol levels. And researchers have also found that dietary fiber may help lower various markers of inflammation in the body (like C-reactive protein), which when elevated may contribute to the development of plaque in the arteries and heart disease. But consuming as little as 12 grams and up to about 33 grams of dietary fiber each day—from whole foods, not supplements—may help lower blood pressure, improve blood cholesterol and triglyceride levels, and reduce inflammation. And chia seeds are an excellent (and simple-to-use) fiber-rich whole food that can help you meet your daily needs. A single ounce meets 30 to 80 percent of the recommended daily intake of dietary fiber for heart health.

Chia Seeds Rich in Cancer-Fighting Antioxidants and Fiber

Boosting your fiber intake with whole foods like chia seeds not only benefits your heart and blood sugars but may also slash your risk of certain types of cancers. Researchers have found that bumping up your intake of fiber-rich foods may lower your risk of mouth, breast, small intestine, and colon cancers. Fiber increases the bulk of the stool, keeping waste matter (including toxins) moving through the intestines and out of the body. In doing so, it limits the contact between potentially cancer-causing substances present in the gut and your intestinal lining. In addition, when fiber is fermented in the colon by the bacteria that reside there, they produce short-chain fatty acids, which researchers believe not only "feed" the cells of the colon, but also exert anticancer properties. These are good reasons to pair chia seeds and other fiber-rich foods with probiotic-rich fermented foods like kefir, kombucha, and sauerkraut.

In addition to fiber, chia seeds are rich in antioxidants like heart-healthy and cancer-fighting flavonoids (including myricetin and quercetin) and cinnamic acids (like caffeic acid). Researchers have found that some of chia's greatest antioxidant activity comes from myricetin, a compound that, in cell studies, has been found to reduce inflammation and exert anticancer properties. It may also help improve blood sugar and triglyceride levels. And in a few recent cell studies, researchers have found that extracts of chia prevent the growth and spreading of certain types of cancers, including those of the breast.

Putting It into Practice

Chia seeds contain a wonderful blend of health-promoting nutrients, including omega-3 fatty acids, dietary fiber, and antioxidants. I have provided a few simple tips to incorporate chia into your diet—along with a few other diet and lifestyle strategies—to support a strong heart and better blood sugars.

- Try adding 1 ounce of chia seeds (2 to 2½ tablespoons, or 25 to 31 g) to your daily diet to give your body the extra 10-gram boost of fiber and other nutrients it needs for optimal weight and health. Incorporate chia into your diet

SPOTLIGHT: ARGININE

Chia seeds are rich in arginine, a heart-healthy amino acid. Arginine is considered a "semi-essential" amino acid, which means that although your body can produce it, you may have increased needs from time to time that can be met by consuming arginine-rich foods—like chia seeds.

In the body, arginine changes into nitric oxide, a chemical that acts as a vasodilator, which helps the blood vessels widen and relax. For this reason, eating foods rich in arginine (or in some cases, taking an L-arginine supplement) may help lower blood pressure or treat certain conditions of the heart, like angina (chest pain), congestive heart failure (CHF), and coronary artery disease. And because it acts on the blood vessels, it may also be useful in the treatment of erectile dysfunction.

In addition to chia seeds, foods rich in arginine include nuts and seeds such as walnuts, almonds, Brazil nuts, and sesame seeds as well as coconut, chocolate, and meat, fish, and poultry. As the nutrients in food tend to work in sync with each other, I almost always recommend whole foods over supplements. But if you choose to take a supplement like L-arginine, be sure to consult with your health care provider first—especially if you are taking any medications.

over the course of the day—a teaspoon or two at a time into freshly pressed juices, blended smoothies, soups, cereals, and salads.

- Experiment with a few of the heart-healthy recipes in this chapter. I've combined the power of chia seeds with superfoods like chocolate, pomegranate, green tea, and blueberries—all known for their high levels of heart-protective antioxidants and phytochemicals. Try the Super Berry Overnight Oatmeal Bowl (page 120) or (Real) Chocolate Lover's Chia Pudding (page 119) for breakfast (yes, chocolate for breakfast!); the Blueberry Chia Granola Bars (page 130) or Lemon, Coconut & Chocolate Chia Bark (page 132) as a between-meal snack; or the Creamy Cauliflower Soup (page 124) or Roasted Brussels Sprouts & Grapes (page 125) for dinner.

- Experiment with a few of the blood sugar–friendly dishes in this chapter. I've combined the power of fiber- and protein-rich chia seeds with other low-glycemic foods and blood sugar–friendly spices (like cinnamon) to take full advantage of their beneficial effects on blood sugars. Try the Hearty Black Bean, Brown Rice, & Root Veggie Patties (page 122) for dinner or the No-Bake Apple & Cinnamon Cookie (page 131) when you are craving a sweet treat.

- Incorporate healthy fats into your diet. In addition to ALA-rich chia seeds, there are other foods that are rich in heart-healthy monounsaturated and poly-unsaturated omega-3 fats, including olives, olive oil, avocados, walnuts, and flaxseeds. You can also enjoy a small amount (about a tablespoon a day) of saturated fats from whole foods like real butter and coconut oil, the latter of which does not appear to have an effect—positive or negative—on cholesterol or triglyceride levels. As a general rule, you should limit your total fat intake to less than 30 percent of your total calories (about 66 grams of total fat on a 2000-calorie diet) and limit your saturated fat intake to less than 10 percent of your total calories (about 20 grams of saturated fat on a 2000-calorie diet—the amount you would find in 2 tablespoons [28 grams] of real butter or about 1½ tablespoons [21 g] of coconut oil).

- Of course, there are other factors—beyond the simple addition of fiber- and omega-3 fat-rich foods like chia seeds—that can improve heart health. Quitting smoking, reducing stress, exercising (even as little as a 30-minute walk each day), and limiting alcohol intake for those who choose to drink (a maximum of two drinks per day for men and one drink per day for women) may all help reduce your risk for heart disease and other chronic diseases.

RECIPES AT A GLANCE

Chia-Inspired Recipes for Health

Sparkling Pomegranate & Blueberry Chia Fresca

Pomegranates and blueberries are super fruits that contain heart-healthy, cancer-fighting compounds. This sparkling beverage combines the sweet juice of fresh blueberries with 100 percent pure pomegranate juice—with a sprinkle of pomegranate arils on the bottom. If you are feeling adventurous (and don't mind the mess), feel free to make juice from fresh pomegranate arils instead of using bottled pomegranate juice.

¼   **cup (44 g) fresh pomegranate arils**
2   **cups (290 g) fresh blueberries (or [310 g] thawed frozen)**
1   **cup (235 ml) pure pomegranate juice**
1   **liter (950 ml) sparkling water, chilled**
2   **tablespoons (25 g) chia seeds**

Place the pomegranate arils in a large pitcher and gently crush to release their juice. Push the blueberries through a juicer and pour the freshly pressed blueberry juice, pure pomegranate juice, and sparkling water into the pitcher. Stir in the chia seeds and let stand for about 10 minutes, stirring once or twice during that time.

Pour into glasses and serve chilled. Refrigerate any unused portion in an airtight container for 2 to 3 days.

Yield: Serves 6 to 8

Cherry & Vanilla Chia Smoothie

This smoothie is a dreamy and creamy combination of unsweetened coconut milk and sweet dark cherries, which are packed with cancer-fighting carotenoids and heart-healthy flavonoids. These super fruits are also known for their ability to help fight inflammation—in fact, they are one of my favorite arthritis-fighting foods. And for those looking to improve sleep quality and quantity, melatonin-rich cherries (especially the tart ones) just might help you catch a few extra z's. Enjoy this super smoothie for super health and well-being.

2   cups (312 g) frozen sweet cherries
1½ cups (355 ml) unsweetened
     coconut milk
1   cup (225) crushed ice
2   teaspoons chia seeds
½   teaspoon pure vanilla extract

Combine all of the ingredients in a high-speed blender and blend until smooth.

Yield: Serves 1 to 2

Minty Jasmine Green Tea & Super Berry Smoothie

The combination of green tea with super berries like blueberries and açai berries makes this sweet and subtly minty smoothie an antioxidant powerhouse. Green tea contains cancer-fighting catechins, and both açai and blueberries are packed with heart-healthy flavonoids called anthocyanins, which give these berries their dark purple color and help relax the body's blood vessels. The compounds in these three power foods are good for the heart, may help destroy certain types of cancer cells, and may even boost brain power.

2   **cups (310 g) frozen blueberries**
1½ **cups (355 ml) brewed jasmine green tea, chilled**
1   **frozen açai berry smoothie pack (100 g)**
1   **tablespoon (12.5 g) chia seeds**
1   **tablespoon (6 g) chopped fresh mint leaves**

Combine all of the ingredients in a high-speed blender and blend until smooth.

Yield: Serves 1 to 2

(Real) Chocolate Lover's Chia Pudding

Antioxidant-rich raw cacao powder is the finely ground powder made from raw cacao beans, the seeds found within the fruits of the cacao tree—and the source of all chocolate. Small amounts of chocolate—especially raw cacao and dark chocolate containing at least 70 percent cacao—are good for the heart and may help boost mood and reduce stress. This easy-to-make, fiber-rich pudding is perfect to have on hand any time you are craving a sweet and chocolaty treat.

2	cups (475 ml) unsweetened coconut milk
6	pitted dates
3	tablespoons (18 g) raw cacao powder
1½	teaspoons pure vanilla extract
½	vanilla bean, scraped, or additional ½ teaspoon pure vanilla extract
½	cup (100 g) chia seeds
¼	cup (32 g) raw cacao nibs
	Pure maple syrup, to taste (optional)

Combine the coconut milk, dates, cacao powder, vanilla extract, and vanilla seeds in a high-speed blender and blend until smooth. Pour into a container with a tight-fitting lid (I like to use a mason jar or Pyrex storage dish), add the chia seeds, and shake. Alternatively, you can pour the liquid into a bowl and stir in the chia seeds to combine. Let the pudding rest for 30 minutes, shaking or stirring every 5 to 10 minutes, until thick.

Pour the pudding into serving bowls, top with cacao nibs, drizzle with maple syrup, and serve.

Yield: Serves 3 or 4

Super Berry Overnight Oatmeal Bowl

Sweet, crunchy, and so tasty, this super berry bowl is the ultimate antioxidant-packed cereal. Fresh and dried super berries, raw cacao nibs, walnuts (which contain one of the highest levels of antioxidants of all nuts), and chia combine in this simple-to-make, hearty breakfast bowl.

1   cup (235 ml) coconut milk
½   cup (40 g) rolled oats (see Note)
¼   cup (25 g) raw walnuts, chopped
1   tablespoon (7 g) sweetened dried cranberries
1   tablespoon (10 g) unsweetened dried tart cherries
1   tablespoon (6 g) goji berries
1   tablespoon (8 g) raw cacao nibs
2   teaspoons chia seeds
¼   cup (about 145 g) fresh seasonal berries (such as blueberries, blackberries, or raspberries)
    Honey, to taste (optional)

Combine the coconut milk, oats, walnuts, cranberries, cherries, goji berries, cacao nibs, and chia seeds in a mason jar or bowl with a tight-fitting lid and shake or stir to combine. Refrigerate overnight.

Pour into a serving bowl, top with fresh berries, drizzle with honey, and serve.

Yield: Serves 1 to 2

Note: This recipe is gluten-free if you use gluten-free rolled oats. Although traditional oats do not contain wheat, barley, or rye (all of which contain gluten), they may become contaminated with these gluten-containing grains during processing. For this reason, if you are following a gluten-free diet, consume only oats labeled "gluten-free."

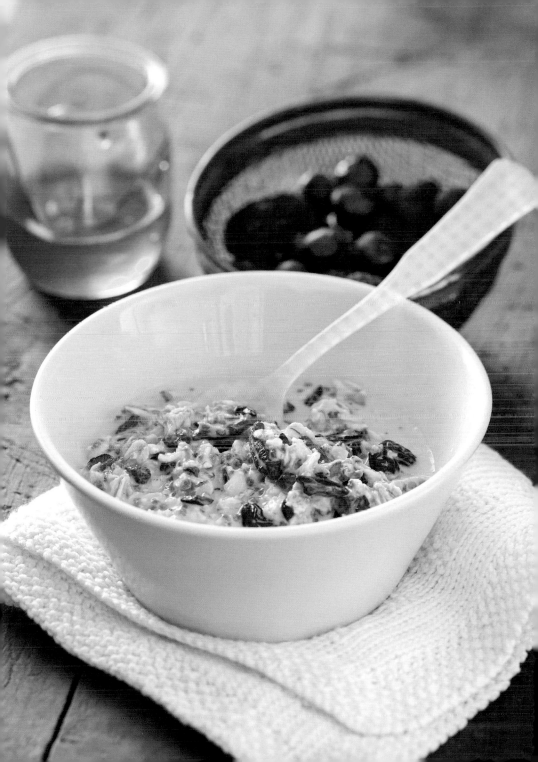

Hearty Black Bean, Brown Rice & Root Veggie Patties

This hearty veggie burger makes it easy to go meatless on Mondays (or any day of the week). The beets in this burger are rich in nitrates, which may help lower blood pressure (nitrates are converted to nitric oxide in the body, which dilates blood vessels and improves blood flow). Enjoy this burger alone or on a slice or two of whole-grain, sprouted-grain, or gluten-free bread with a spread of Garlicky Chia Hummus (page 40), Avocado Chia Mash (page 126), or Fiery Chia Guacamole (page 152).

1   can (15 ounces, or 425 g) black beans, rinsed and drained

1   cup (195 g) cooked brown rice

¼   cup (50 g) chia seeds

1   medium onion, diced

1   medium red beet, peeled and diced

1   large carrot, peeled and diced

3   cloves garlic, crushed

2   tablespoons (8 g) chopped fresh parsley

1   tablespoon (15 ml) extra-virgin olive oil

   Sea salt and freshly ground black pepper, to taste

2   large eggs, beaten

2   tablespoons (17 g) Bob's Red Mill all-purpose gluten-free baking flour

1   tablespoon (15 ml) canola oil, plus more for browning (preferably organic, expeller pressed)

Place the black beans in a large bowl and mash with a fork. Add the rice, chia seeds, onion, beet, carrot, garlic, parsley, and olive oil and stir until combined. Season with sea salt and black pepper. Add the eggs and flour and mix well.

Heat the canola oil in a large skillet over medium-high heat. Form each patty by very tightly packing together ½ cup (115 g) of the filling. Place the patties onto the skillet, in batches if necessary, and cook until brown and cooked through, 6 to 8 minutes on each side. Serve warm.

Yield: 6 to 8 patties

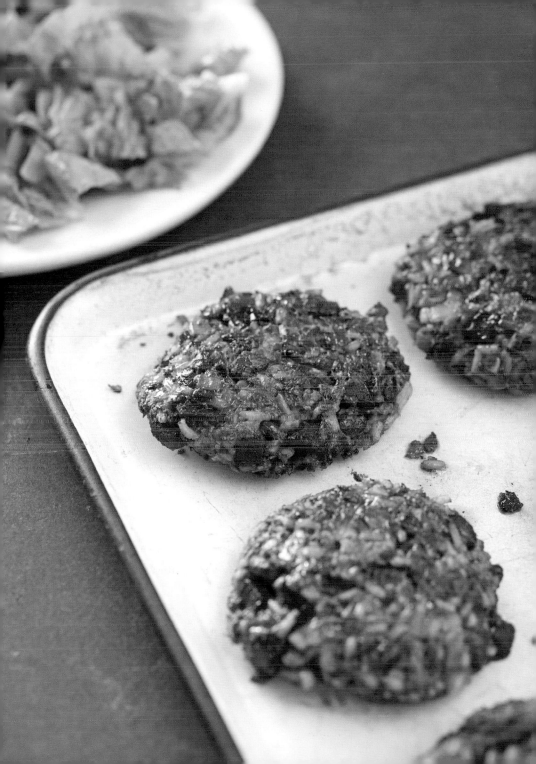

Creamy Cauliflower Soup

Cauliflower, a cruciferous vegetable that is packed with cancer-fighting glucosinolates, forms the base of this thick and creamy soup. Pine nuts and crushed garlic add subtle flavor, while the fiber-rich milled chia seeds give a little boost of fiber and work as a thickener—resulting in a heart-healthy, creamy soup. Top with your choice of nutritional yeast or Parmesan cheese.

1 tablespoon (15 ml) extra-virgin olive oil

½ medium onion, finely chopped

3 cloves garlic, crushed, divided

1 large head cauliflower, florets removed

4 cups (950 ml) vegetable broth

⅓ cup (45 g) pine nuts

1 tablespoon (12.5 g) milled chia seeds

Sea salt and freshly ground black pepper, to taste

Nutritional yeast or Parmesan cheese (optional), for serving

Heat the oil in a large pot over medium heat. Add the onion and 2 cloves of the crushed garlic and sauté until soft, about 3 minutes.

Add the cauliflower and vegetable broth to the pot (the broth will just barely cover the cauliflower) and bring to a boil. Reduce the heat, cover, and simmer for 20 to 30 minutes, stirring occasionally, until the florets are soft and tender.

Remove from the heat and stir in the pine nuts, milled chia seeds, and the remaining 1 clove crushed garlic. Blend with an immersion blender until smooth and creamy. (If you do not have an immersion blender, let the soup cool, puree in small batches in a high-speed blender, and return to the pot.) Season with sea salt and black pepper. Pour into serving bowls, top with a sprinkle of nutritional yeast or Parmesan cheese, and serve warm.

Yield: Serves 4 to 6

Roasted Brussels Sprouts & Grapes

Roasting vegetables is so incredibly easy. Toss your favorite vegetables with a little extra-virgin olive oil, season with salt and pepper, and pop in the oven—so simple! In this recipe, I combine Brussels sprouts, one of the richest sources of cancer-fighting glucosinolates (even more than cauliflower, kale, and broccoli), with grapes, an antioxidant-packed super fruit whose beneficial polyphenols may improve heart health. Toss these mini cabbages and sweet fruits with a few generous spoonfuls of chia seeds for extra fiber, fat, and protein.

2	pounds (910 g) Brussels sprouts
3	tablespoons (45 ml) extra-virgin olive oil
	Sea salt and freshly ground black pepper, to taste
1½	pounds (680 g) red grapes
2	tablespoons (25 g) chia seeds

Preheat the oven to 400°F (200°C, or gas mark 6).

Trim the ends of the Brussels sprouts, remove and discard any wilted or browned outer leaves, and halve. Place the Brussels sprouts in a large bowl, drizzle with the olive oil, season with sea salt and black pepper, and toss to combine.

Transfer the Brussels sprouts to a large roasting pan and roast for 20 to 25 minutes, stirring occasionally. Add the grapes and roast for an additional 20 to 25 minutes, stirring occasionally, until the Brussels sprouts are browned.

Remove from the oven and toss with the chia seeds. Serve warm.

Yield: Serves 6 to 8

Open-Face PLT Sandwiches with Avocado Chia Mash

The "P" in PLT stands for parsnip, a sweet root vegetable that is a relative of the carrot. A few years ago, I read about a "parsnip bacon" trend in *Food & Wine* magazine. I fell in love with the salty crunch of the "bacon" and began using it in sandwiches (when I wasn't devouring the crunchy crisps alone). Top this sandwich with a generous spread of Avocado Chia Mash for flavor and health.

1   parsnip
1   tablespoon (15 ml) extra-virgin olive oil
    Sea salt, to taste
1   avocado, halved, pitted, and peeled
1/2 teaspoon freshly squeezed lime juice
1   teaspoon chia seeds
4   slices whole-grain, sprouted-grain, or gluten-free bread of choice
4   leaves romaine lettuce
1   medium tomato, sliced

Preheat the oven to 300°F (150°C, or gas mark 2). Peel the parsnip lengthwise into wide, thin strips using a vegetable peeler. Lay the parsnip strips on a baking sheet lined with parchment paper. Brush the olive oil on both sides of the parsnip strips and season with sea salt. Place a sheet of parchment paper over the parsnips and cover the pan with another baking sheet so that the parsnip strips are firmly pressed between the pans. Bake for about 40 minutes until the parsnip strips are golden brown and crisp.

In a small bowl, combine the avocado halves, lime juice, chia seeds, and pinch of sea salt and mash. Spread about 1 tablespoon (15 g) (or more) of the mash onto each slice of bread. Top with a lettuce leaf, a slice or two of tomato, and a few strips of parsnip bacon and serve.

Yield: Serves 4

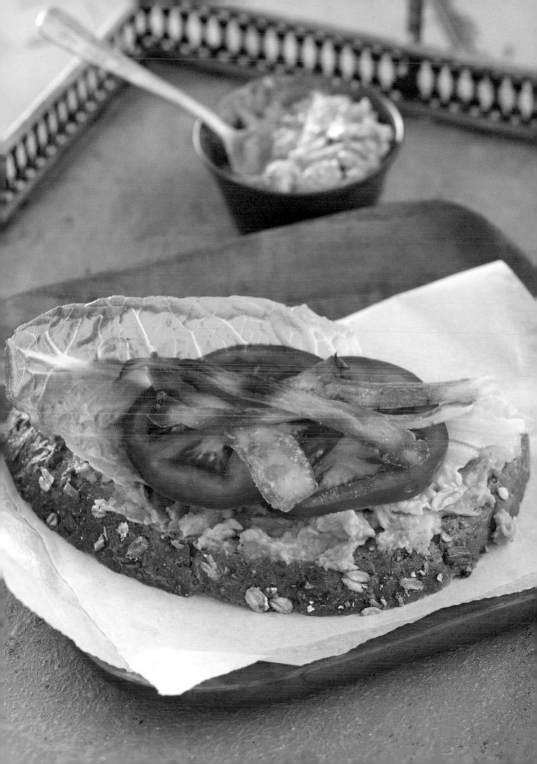

Chunky Garlic & Cilantro Chia Salsa

This chunky salsa is packed with flavorful cilantro and fresh, raw garlic. Rich in beneficial sulfur-containing compounds, garlic may help lower blood pressure and total and LDL ("bad") cholesterol. In fact, researchers have found that including just 1 clove of garlic in the diet each day may help lower blood pressure by as much as 7 to 8 percent.

2   cups (360 g) chopped tomatoes

½   cup (8 g) chopped fresh cilantro

¼   cup (40 g) finely chopped red onion

2 or 3 cloves garlic, crushed

2   tablespoons (25 g) chia seeds

1   tablespoon (15 ml) extra-virgin olive oil

1   tablespoon (15 ml) freshly squeezed lime juice

Sea salt, to taste

Combine all of the ingredients in a large bowl, let stand for 30 minutes until thick, and serve, or refrigerate until ready to serve.

Yield: 2½ cups (325 g)

Spiced Maple & Cranberry Chia Pecans

This sweet and spicy mix is a delightful treat during the fall and winter months. Pecans are rich in heart-healthy fats, contain a diverse array of vitamins and minerals, and like walnuts boast one of the highest levels of antioxidants of all nuts. Enjoy a handful of this mix any time you are craving something crunchy and sweet.

¼ **cup plus 2 tablespoons (120 g) pure maple syrup**

½ **teaspoon ground cinnamon**

   Pinch of ground nutmeg

   Pinch of ground cloves

   Pinch of sea salt

2 **cups (200 g) raw pecan halves**

½ **cup (60 g) sweetened dried cranberries, chopped**

¼ **cup (50 g) chia seeds**

Preheat the oven to 325°F (170°C, or gas mark 3). In a large bowl, whisk together the maple syrup, cinnamon, nutmeg, cloves, and sea salt. Stir in the pecans, cranberries, and chia seeds and toss until the nuts are well coated. Transfer the mixture to a large baking sheet and bake for 15 minutes, stirring occasionally.

Transfer the mixture to a piece of waxed paper and let cool completely. Store in an airtight container or bag. This keeps best refrigerated or frozen.

Yield: About 3 cups (255 g)

Blueberry Chia Granola Bars

Antioxidant-packed blueberries, protein-rich super seeds (like hemp and chia), and calcium- and fiber-rich almonds star in this chewy dehydrated bar, which is lightly sweetened with a touch of agave syrup, a sweetener with a low glycemic index. Blueberries are good for the heart, and researchers have found that eating 2 cups (290 g) of blueberries a week may lower your risk of diabetes by 25 percent.

2	cups (290 g) fresh blueberries
1	cup (145 g) raw almonds, chopped
1/2	cup (160 g) agave syrup
1/4	cup (50 g) chia seeds
1/4	cup (30 g) hemp seeds
1/4	cup (36 g) raw sunflower seeds
1	teaspoon lemon zest
1/2	teaspoon pure vanilla extract
	Pinch of sea salt

Place all of the ingredients in a food processor and briefly pulse 6 or 8 times into a moist, thick, and chunky mixture, being careful not to overprocess. Transfer the mixture to a Teflex-lined dehydrator tray and using a spatula, spread the mixture into an approximately 10-inch (25 cm) square that's 1/2 inch (1 cm) thick. Dehydrate at 105°F (41°C) for about 24 hours until dry to the touch but still soft.

Remove the tray from the dehydrator and carefully slide the Teflex sheet off of the dehydrator screen. Flip the granola over onto a dry cutting board and gently peel the Teflex sheet off. Cut the granola into 2 1/2 x 5-inch (6 x 13 cm) bars and place the individual bars directly on the mesh screen (you may need to use a spatula to transfer the bars).

Continue to dehydrate the bars at 105°F (41°C) for an additional 8 to 10 hours. The granola bars are done when they are firm, dry, and slightly chewy. Store in an airtight container.

Yield: 8 bars

No-Bake Apple & Cinnamon Cookies

These flourless cookies are a favorite in our home. They effortlessly combine prebiotic-rich apples (with their peel, which contains more than a dozen different cancer-fighting compounds), omega-3 fatty acid–rich walnuts and chia seeds, fiber-rich raisins, and blood sugar–balancing cinnamon. In fact, cinnamon is thought to have the most positive effect on blood sugars of all spices, and it seems that as little as ½ teaspoon per day may be all that is needed to help balance them.

5   medium apples, cored and chopped
1   teaspoon freshly squeezed
    lemon juice
1½ cups (150 g) raw walnuts, chopped
1½ cups (220 g) raisins
½   cup (160 g) agave syrup
3   tablespoons (37.5 g) chia seeds
2   tablespoons (14 g) ground cinnamon

In a large bowl, toss the apples with the lemon juice. Stir in the walnuts, raisins, agave syrup, chia seeds, and cinnamon. Shape tightly packed 2-tablespoon-size (28 g) scoops of cookie "dough" into a ball (I use a #40 scoop), place onto a mesh dehydrator screen, and gently flatten. Dehydrate at 105°F (41°C) for about 12 hours for a soft and chewy cookie. Store in an airtight container.

Yield: About 30 cookies

Lemon, Coconut & Chocolate Chia Bark

This is an incredibly simple and decadent sweet treat combining smooth and creamy dark chocolate with crunchy chia seeds, dried coconut, and lemon zest. I like to use dark chocolate chips, which have a higher percentage of heart-healthy cacao than other varieties, but feel free to use your favorite chip, including nondairy chocolate chips or carob chips.

1   **bag (9 ounces, or 255 g) dark chocolate chips**
½   **cup (43 g) shredded dried coconut**
¼   **cup (50 g) chia seeds**
1   **tablespoon (6 g) lemon zest**
    Pinch of sea salt

Melt the chocolate chips in a small saucepan over medium heat, stirring occasionally, until smooth and creamy. Remove from the heat and stir in the dried coconut, chia seeds, and lemon zest. Spread the thick mixture into an even layer on a baking sheet lined with waxed paper. Freeze until hard, about 30 minutes.

Break into bite-size chunks. Store in an airtight container.

Yield: About 24 pieces

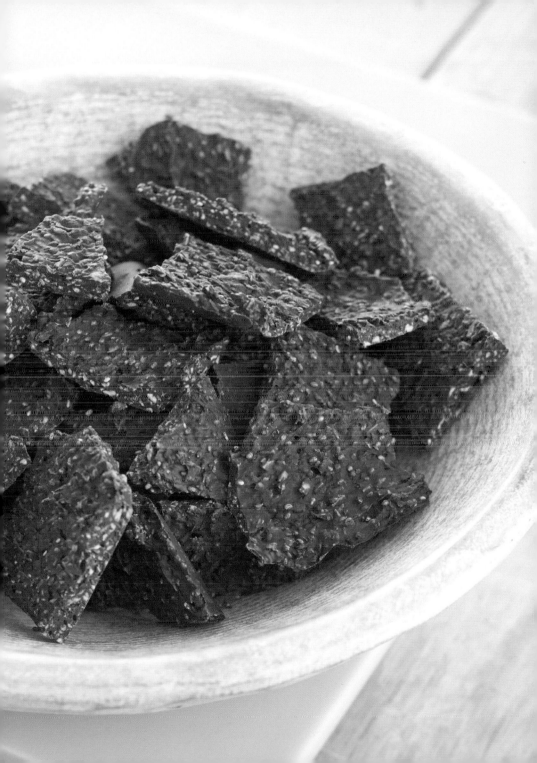

CHAPTER 5

Get Glowing: Omega-3 Fat–Rich Chia For Beauty

As an adolescent, I went to my dermatologist to help treat what was a fairly harsh case of acne. Following at least three rounds of different types of antibiotics and a dizzying array of drying ointments and sulfur-based (and stinky!) topical creams, my mother finally asked the dermatologist if there was anything in my diet I could change to help improve my complexion. His answer: that diet had absolutely nothing to do with the state of my skin—unless I was to touch my face while eating greasy food like chips or pizza, of course. And that was that. So I went on a course of a strong prescription medication for acne that I would years later find out carries severe warnings for side effects ranging from chapped lips to increased risk of suicide. And years later, I would also discover that diet does, indeed, affect the health of the skin.

Fortunately, times have changed. What happens inside your body is reflected outside your body on your largest organ: your skin. And doctors are finding that both what you put in your body and what you put on your skin has a tremendous impact on skin health. In this chapter, we'll explore some of the beneficial nutrients in chia seeds—namely, their essential fatty acids—that may help boost the health of your skin. I'll share with you a few ways to use chia topically in a few recipes for fun and effective face masks, courtesy of my favorite green beauty experts. And in the recipes in this chapter, I'll show you how to amp up the power of chia seeds by combining them with some of my favorite beautifying foods, like cucumbers, coconut oil, pineapples, greens, and berries, to leave you glowing inside and out!

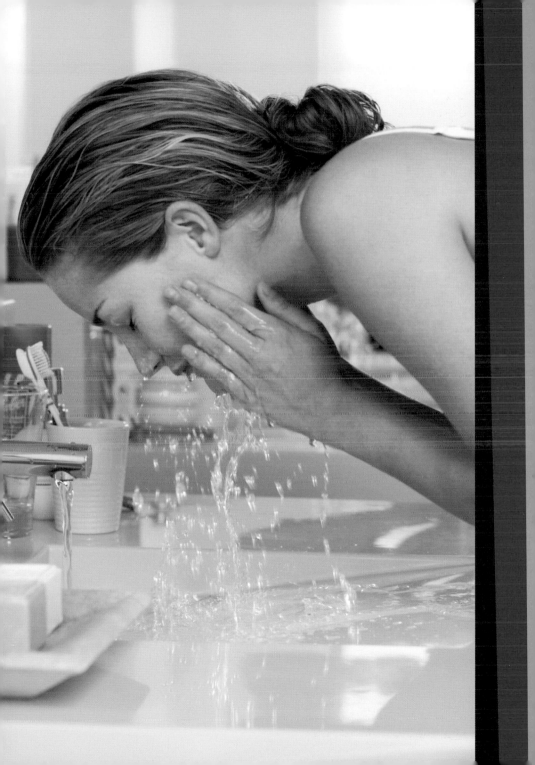

Fat- and Mineral-Rich Chia Seeds for Healthy Skin

Chia seeds are an excellent source of the skin-protecting, plant-based omega-3 fatty acid alpha-linolenic acid (ALA). Researchers have found that omega-3 fatty acids like ALA may help reduce inflammation in the skin (and other parts of the body), prevent sunburn, promote wound healing, and maintain the outermost surface of the skin. In addition, they may help promote the destruction of certain cancerous cells, including melanoma skin cancers. Indeed, reports indicate that the ancient Aztecs used the oil from chia seeds on the skin. Today, researchers are finding that the fats from omega-3 fatty acid–rich foods may protect against or ease the symptoms associated with a number of skin conditions ranging from acne and dry skin to eczema and psoriasis. In one small study published in 2010, researchers noted significant improvements in the health of the skin in 10 patients with symptoms of pruritis and xerosis (which is simply abnormally dry and itchy skin) after using a topical 4 percent chia seed oil for 8 weeks.

The fat in chia seeds also helps the body absorb important fat-soluble vitamins like vitamins A and E, both of which are antioxidant vitamins that help protect cells (including skin cells) against free radical damage and may help prevent breakouts and dryness. And chia seeds, in particular, are also a good source of skin-supporting minerals like zinc, which researchers have found to be effective against certain skin conditions like acne and dandruff. Chia seeds contain over 1 milligram of zinc per ounce—about 10 percent of the average adult's daily needs. Other good sources include pumpkin seeds and Brazil nuts, which I have incorporated into the recipes in this chapter.

Putting It into Practice

Implement one or more of the following tips to leave your complexion soft, supple, and glowing. And then get started experimenting with some of the recipes that follow—including a few facial mask recipes!

- Try adding 2 to 3 teaspoons (8 to 12.5 g) of chia seeds to your daily diet. This amount supplies the much-needed inflammation-fighting, skin-soothing, omega-3 fatty acid alpha-linolenic acid. You can toss chia into freshly pressed juices and smoothies or onto salads or experiment with some of the beautifying recipes in this section—like the Carrot & Pineapple Smoothie (page 146) or the Creamy Pumpkin Pie Chia Pudding (page 149)—that combine the omega-3 power of chia seeds with the antioxidant- and mineral-rich power of a few of my favorite skin-friendly superfoods.

- Drink more water. Prevent dehydrated skin by increasing your water intake. Aim to drink anywhere from 1 to 2 liters (1 to 2 quarts) of pure water each day—in addition to the fluids you take in from sparkling water, freshly pressed juices, smoothies, and water-rich fruits and vegetables.

- Eat more fiber. A boost in fiber can help relieve a sluggish digestive tract—and improve the skin. Adding 2 to 3 teaspoons (8 to 12.5 g) of chia seeds (or up to 2 to 3 tablespoons, or 25 to 37.5 grams) is a great way to boost your fiber intake to the recommended 25 to 35 grams per day. As you may recall from previous chapters, 1 ounce of chia seeds (2 to 2½ tablespoons, or 25 to 31 grams) provides nearly 10 grams of dietary fiber.

- Reduce the sugar and dairy in your diet. When it comes to the food you eat, researchers have found that there may be an association between sugar and dairy intake and acne. These foods seem to promote inflammation, which accelerates aging and can cause acne flare-ups. If you are looking to clear your complexion, try eliminating the "white foods" from your diet (and I don't mean whole foods like cauliflower, potatoes, and bananas), like milk, cheese, yogurt, and products made from white flour, including bread, pasta, cookies, and other baked goods.

- Get enough rest. Keep your complexion glowing with adequate sleep. Everyone is different, but most individuals need 7 to 9 hours of sleep each night. Try gentle stretching or yoga, a warm bath, or essential oils like lavender to wind down and prepare for a good night's sleep.

- Go organic for beauty. There are several wonderful skin care brands that are raw, certified organic, or created without the use of some of the more commonly used toxic skin care ingredients. Some of my favorite brands are Éminence Organic Skin Care (www.eminenceorganics.com), Dr. Alkaitis (www.alkaitis.com), and Dr. Hauschka (www.drhauschka.com). You can find these and similar skin care and makeup lines through online retailers like Saffron Rouge (www.saffronrouge.com) or Spirit Beauty Lounge (www.spiritbeautylounge.com). You can also experiment with the three chia-based facial cleansers and masks I have included at the end of this chapter—courtesy of three of my favorite green beauty experts. Try the Gentle Chia Facial Scrub & Cleanser (page 159), Rejuvenating Chia Face Mask (page 160), or Soothing Chia Beauty Mask (page 161)—good enough to both eat and slather on your skin!

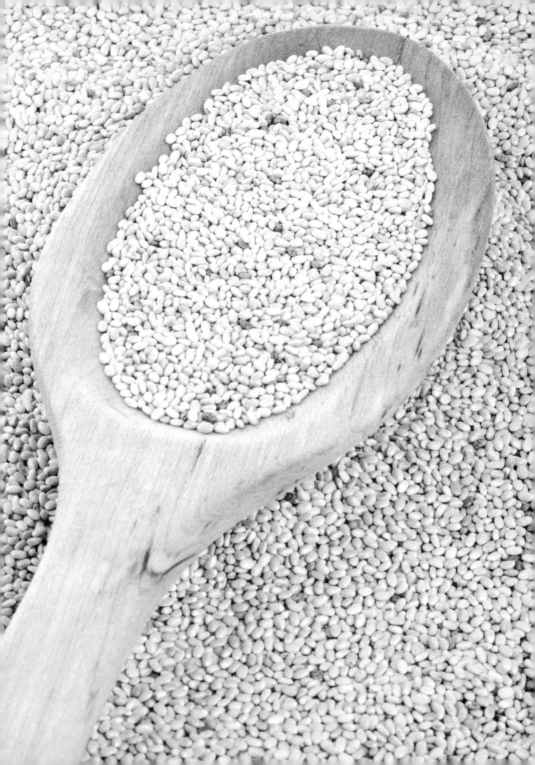

Chia-Inspired Recipes for Beauty

- Green Grapefruit Chia Fresca 141
- Carrot & Pineapple Smoothie 142
- Vanilla, Cashew, & Brazil Nut Milk 144
- Simple Cucumber Chia Elixir 145
- Lavender, Chamomile & Pineapple Chia Elixir 146
- Gingery Vanilla Green Smoothie 148
- Creamy Pumpkin Pie Chia Pudding 149
- Açai Berry Chia Pudding Bowl 151
- Fiery Chia Guacamole 152
- Garlicky Chia Kale Chips 153
- Cinnamon & Spice Sweet Potato Crisps 154
- Pomegranate & Lime Chia Fruit Leather 156
- Lemony Chia Date Balls 157
- Green Tea & Goji Berry Granola Bars 158
- Gentle Chia Facial Scrub & Cleanser 159
- Rejuvenating Chia Face Mask 160
- Soothing Chia Beauty Mask 161

Green Grapefruit Chia Fresca

Grapefruit and green juice are great together—in terms of both taste and nutrition. The tangy and subtly sweet flavor of vitamin C–rich grapefruit is well matched with the alkalizing green juice from chlorophyll-rich wheatgrass. Juicing fresh wheatgrass requires a specialized wheatgrass juicer. If you don't have one, you can buy fresh wheatgrass juice from your local juice bar or health food store or purchase frozen cubes of freshly pressed wheatgrass juice from the freezer section of your local market—a simple and convenient way to get a daily dose of beautifying greens!

2　grapefruits

¼　cup (60 ml) wheatgrass juice (freshly pressed or thawed frozen)

1　teaspoon freshly squeezed lime juice

2　teaspoons chia seeds

　　Honey, to taste (optional)

Squeeze the grapefruit using a citrus press or peel the grapefruit and push through a juicer (they should yield about 1½ cups [355 ml] of juice). Combine the grapefruit, wheatgrass, and lime juices, chia seeds, and honey in a jar with a tight-fitting lid (I like to use a mason jar) and shake to combine. Let stand for about 10 minutes, shaking once or twice.

Serve chilled. Refrigerate any unused portion in an airtight container for 2 to 3 days.

Yield: Serves 1 to 2

Carrot & Pineapple Smoothie

The beta-carotene from carrots and the anti-inflammatory enzymes in pineapple combine with omega-3 fatty acid–rich chia seeds in a creamy cashew and Brazil nut milk base to make a wonderfully beautifying beverage. Brazil nuts, which are packed with skin-soothing and free-radical–fighting selenium are one of my top food picks for skin health. In fact, 1 ounce contains over 500 micrograms of selenium—nearly 800 percent of your daily needs.

2 cups (475 ml) Vanilla, Cashew, & Brazil Nut Milk (recipe follows on page 144)

1 cup (130 g) chopped carrots

1 cup (187 g) frozen pineapple chunks

1 medium banana, peeled

2 teaspoons chia seeds

Combine all of the ingredients in a high-speed blender and blend until smooth.

Yield: Serves 1 to 2

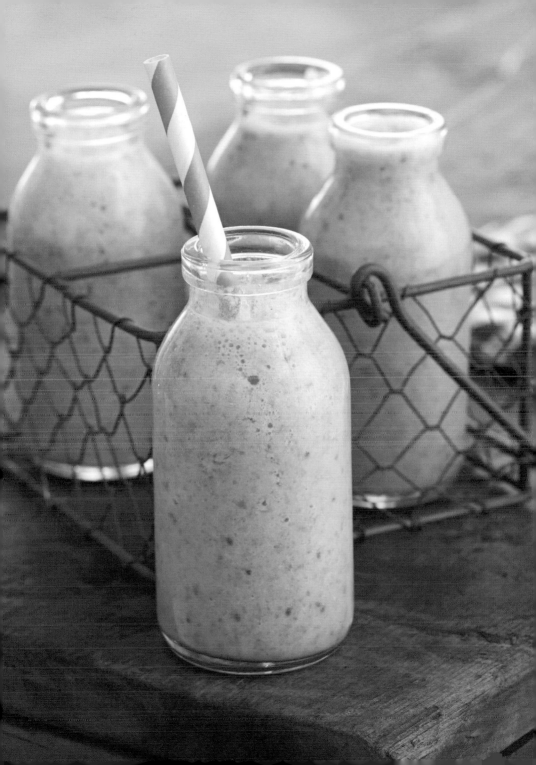

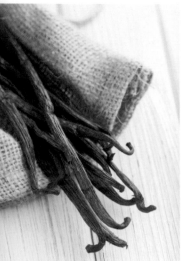 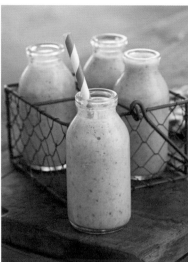 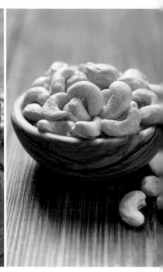

Vanilla, Cashew, & Brazil Nut Milk

½   cup (70 g) raw cashews, soaked in water for 3 to 4 hours

½   cup (67 g) raw Brazil nuts, soaked in water for 3 to 4 hours

4   cups (950 ml) water

4   pitted dates

1   tablespoon (15 ml) coconut oil, melted

1   tablespoon (15 ml) pure vanilla extract

½   vanilla bean, scraped, or additional ½ teaspoon pure vanilla extract

Drain and rinse the cashews and Brazil nuts. Blend the nuts and the water in a high-speed blender for approximately 1 minute. Strain the milk into a separate pitcher using a nut milk bag or strainer. Rinse the blender container with water and return the strained milk to it. Add the remaining ingredients and blend until smooth. Pour into a glass jar with a tight-fitting lid and refrigerate until ready to use. Shake well before serving.

Yield: 4 cups (950 ml)

Simple Cucumber Chia Elixir

Cucumber is one of my favorite beautifying foods, rich in skin-building silica and with a mild diuretic power that can help revive a puffy face and bloated body. I love the refreshing taste of cucumber juice without any added sugar, but if you need to sweeten this juice up, try adding a small spoonful of honey or sweetener of your choice.

2   large cucumbers (peeled if
    not organic)
1   teaspoon freshly squeezed lime juice
2   teaspoons chia seeds
    Honey, to taste (optional)

Push the cucumbers through a juicer (they should yield 1½ to 2 cups [355 to 475 ml] of juice). Combine the cucumber and lime juices, chia seeds, and honey in a jar with a tight-fitting lid (I like to use a mason jar) and shake to combine. Let stand for about 10 minutes, shaking once or twice.

Serve chilled. Refrigerate any unused portion in an airtight container for 2 to 3 days.

Yield: Serves 1 to 2

Lavender, Chamomile & Pineapple Chia Elixir

Beat age-accelerating and acne-causing stress with a combination of soothing lavender and chamomile tea and the beautifying power of pineapple, which is rich in the inflammation-fighting enzyme bromelain. I enjoy brewing a lavender-chamomile tea from one of my favorite tea companies, Traditional Medicinals, but feel free to use any of your favorite brands of bagged or loose-leaf tea. Enjoy this subtly sweet and relaxing elixir any time of day—especially when you want to rest and release stress.

2   cups (330 g) fresh chopped fresh pineapple (or [374 g] thawed frozen)

1½ cups (355 ml) brewed lavender-chamomile tea, chilled

½   vanilla bean, scraped, or ½ teaspoon pure vanilla extract

2   teaspoons chia seeds

Push the chopped pineapple through a juicer (it should yield about 1 cup [235 ml] of juice). Combine the pineapple juice, tea, vanilla seeds or extract, and chia seeds in a jar with a tight-fitting lid (I like to use a mason jar) and shake to combine. Let stand for about 10 minutes, shaking once or twice.

Serve chilled. Refrigerate any unused portion in an airtight container for 2 to 3 days.

Yield: Serves 1 to 2

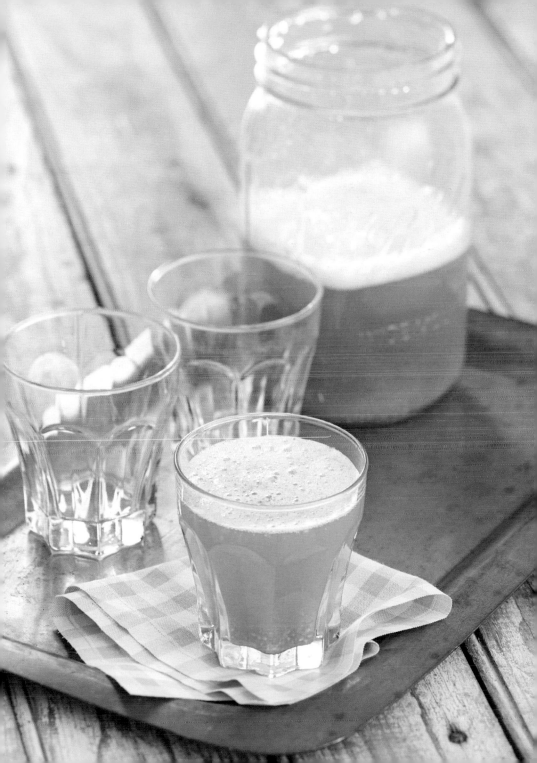

Gingery Vanilla Green Smoothie

This creamy green smoothie combines refreshing cucumbers and sweet pears with the subtle flavors of vanilla, inflammation-quelling ginger, and beautifying coconut oil, whose antimicrobial properties make it an ideal natural moisturizer that can also be applied topically. I like to use sweet and juicy d'Anjou pears for juicing and smoothies, but you can use almost any variety. If they are not yet ripe or sweet enough, you can add a little honey or agave syrup for extra sweetness.

1½ cups (355 ml) unsweetened coconut milk

2 cups (455 g) crushed ice

2 pears, cored and chopped

1 medium cucumber, sliced (peeled if not organic)

1 (2-inch, or 5 cm) piece fresh ginger, peeled and grated

1 tablespoon (12.5 g) chia seeds

1 tablespoon (15 ml) coconut oil, melted

½ teaspoon pure vanilla extract

Honey, to taste (optional)

Combine all of the ingredients in a high-speed blender and blend until smooth.

Yield: Serves 2

Creamy Pumpkin Pie Chia Pudding

This easy-to-assemble pudding combines the fall flavors of beautifying and acne-defying vitamin A–rich pumpkin puree with blood sugar–balancing cinnamon, inflammation-fighting ginger, and other warming spices. It is perfect for breakfast, snack time, or any time you need an immune system– and skin-boosting serving of antioxidants.

2   cups (475 ml) unsweetened coconut milk

1   cup (245 g) pure pumpkin puree

6 to 8 pitted dates

1   teaspoon ground cinnamon

½   teaspoon ground ginger

¼   teaspoon ground nutmeg
      Pinch of ground cloves

½   teaspoon pure vanilla extract

⅓   cup (66.5 g) chia seeds

¼   cup (21 g) shredded dried coconut

Combine the coconut milk, pumpkin puree, dates, cinnamon, ginger, nutmeg, cloves, and vanilla extract in a high-speed blender and blend until smooth. Pour into a container with a tight-fitting lid (I like to use a mason jar or Pyrex storage dish), add the chia seeds, and shake. Alternatively, you can pour the liquid into a separate bowl and stir in the chia seeds to combine. Let the pudding rest for 30 minutes, shaking or stirring every 5 to 10 minutes, until thick.

Pour the pudding into serving bowls, top with the coconut, and serve.

Yield: Serves 3 or 4

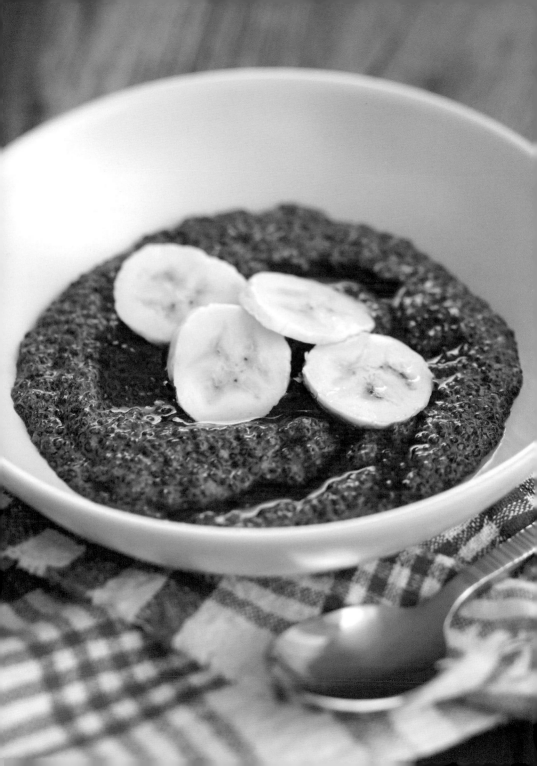

Açai Berry Chia Pudding Bowl

Açai berries are a super berry of the Amazon. In *Powerful Plant-Based Superfoods* (Fair Winds Press, 2013), I describe them as an "antiaging berry for beauty and brains." These superstars are rich in skin-protecting antioxidants and fats like oleic acid, the same monounsaturated fat found in olives and avocados. You can find frozen pouches of pureed açai berries at most supermarkets and health food stores, which you can thaw and blend into this creamy pudding.

1   **cup (235 ml) unsweetened coconut milk**

1   **frozen açai berry smoothie pack (100 g), thawed**

¼   **cup (50 g) chia seeds**

1   **medium banana, sliced**

Agave syrup, to taste (optional)

Combine the coconut milk, açai berry smoothie pack, and chia seeds in a container with a tight-fitting lid (I like to use a mason jar or Pyrex storage dish) and shake. Alternatively, you can combine the coconut milk and açai berry smoothie pack in a bowl and stir in the chia seeds to combine. Let the pudding rest for 30 minutes, shaking or stirring every 5 to 10 minutes, until thick.

Pour the pudding into serving bowls, top with the banana slices, drizzle with agave syrup, and serve.

Yield: Serves 2

Fiery Chia Guacamole

Avocados take center stage in this thick, rich, and spicy guacamole. Avocados are a superfood for the skin, packed with heart- and skin-healthy monounsaturated fats (the same fats found in olive oil) and skin-protecting carotenoids. A sprinkle of chia seeds not only helps to thicken this delicious dip but also provides an added boost of healthy fats and fiber.

2   avocados, halved, pitted, and peeled

¼   cup (60 ml) freshly squeezed lime juice

3   scallions, finely chopped

1   jalapeño pepper, seeded and pith removed

½   cup (8 g) fresh cilantro, finely chopped

2   teaspoons chia seeds

Sea salt, to taste

In a medium bowl, mash the avocado with the lime juice using a potato masher or fork. Stir in the scallions, jalapeño, cilantro, and chia seeds. Season with sea salt and serve.

If preparing in advance, you can help prevent browning by storing the guacamole in a small bowl and covering the top with plastic wrap, pressing the wrap directly onto the top of the guacamole. If the top layer should brown, simply scrape off the top layer, fluff the guacamole with a fork, and serve.

Yield: 1½ to 2 cups (355 to 450 g)

Garlicky Chia Kale Chips

Say good-bye to processed foods—including bagged chips—
that can leave you with a lackluster complexion. These crunchy
kale chips are packed with beneficial vitamins, minerals, and
antioxidants (like bone-building vitamin K and calcium and skin-
boosting beta-carotene) as well as skin-soothing omega-3 fatty
acids from chia. They are a perfect snack for those times when you
are craving a savory and crispy treat. They are best enjoyed fresh,
within 2 to 3 days of preparing—if they last that long. You will need
a food dehydrator for this recipe.

1	large bunch curly kale
1	cup (140 g) raw cashews, soaked in water for 3 to 4 hours
2	tablespoons (28 ml) freshly squeezed lemon juice
1	clove garlic, crushed
¼	teaspoon sea salt
	Freshly ground black pepper, to taste
2	tablespoons (25 g) chia seeds

Remove the tough kale stems, chop the leaves into 2- to 3-inch (5 to 7.5 cm) pieces, and transfer to a large bowl.

Drain and rinse the cashews. In a food processor, combine the cashews, lemon juice, garlic, sea salt, and black pepper. Process until a thick paste forms, stopping to scrape down the sides of the container as needed. Add the cashew paste and chia seeds to the bowl with the kale. Using your fingertips, begin to massage the kale leaves with the mixture until the leaves are evenly coated. Place the kale leaves on the dehydrator screens in a single layer and dehydrate at 105 to 110°F (41 to 43°C) for 2 to 3 hours until crisp. Store in an airtight container. Avoid storing in a plastic bag, as they will soften and crumble.

Yield: About 6 cups (420 g)

Cinnamon & Spice Sweet Potato Crisps

These chips are a sweet, spicy, and crispy treat. Sweet potatoes are rich in cancer-fighting, immune-boosting, and skin-soothing carotenoids like beta-carotene, which are converted to vitamin A in the body. In fact, one medium sweet potato meets more than 400 percent of your daily vitamin A needs. Warming spices like cinnamon and ginger add flavor and also help ease inflammation. Enjoy these chips any time you are craving a sweet and crunchy snack.

3   **medium sweet potatoes (about 1 pound, or 455 g)**

3   **tablespoons (45 ml) extra-virgin olive oil**

2   **tablespoons (25 g) chia seeds**

1   **teaspoon ground cinnamon**

½   **teaspoon ground ginger**

¼   **teaspoon ground nutmeg**

Pinch of ground cloves

Few pinches of sea salt

Preheat the oven to 300°F (150°C, or gas mark 2). Peel the potatoes and slice into paper-thin disks (I use a mandoline). In a large bowl, toss the potato disks with the olive oil and chia seeds. In a small bowl, stir together the cinnamon, ginger, nutmeg, and cloves. Arrange the chips in a single layer on 2 or 3 large rimmed baking sheets. Sprinkle the seasonings evenly over the chips and season with a few pinches of sea salt. Bake for 20 to 25 minutes, flipping the chips about halfway through the cooking time, until crisp.

Yield: 5 to 6 cups (125 to 150 g)

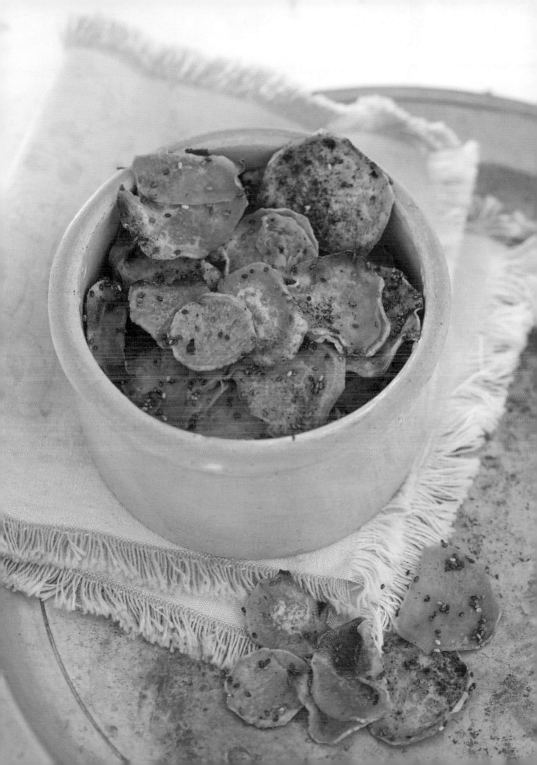

Pomegranate & Lime Chia Fruit Leather

These chewy-crunchy strips provide a simple way to get a big boost of fiber and skin-soothing omega-3 fatty acids from chia seeds, along with the antioxidant power of pomegranate juice and lime. Enjoy as a sweet between-meal snack or before, during, or after your workout. They are easy to pack and enjoy on the go.

1	cup (235 ml) pure pomegranate juice
2	teaspoons freshly squeezed lime juice
½	cup (50 g) chia seeds

Combine all of the ingredients in a container with a tight-fitting lid (I like to use a mason jar or Pyrex storage container) and shake. Let the mixture rest for 30 minutes, stirring or shaking every 5 to 10 minutes, until a thick gel forms.

Using a spatula, spread the gel on a Teflex-lined dehydrator sheet in a very thin layer. Use the edge of the spatula to shape the gel into a large square, which should cover more than three-quarters of the sheet. Dehydrate at 105°F (41°C) for about 3½ hours.

Remove the tray from the dehydrator and carefully slide the Teflex sheet off of the dehydrator screen. Flip the fruit leather over onto the mesh screen and gently peel the Teflex sheet off of the fruit leather. Place the tray back in the dehydrator and continue to dehydrate at 105°F (41°C) for an additional 30 minutes. The fruit leather is done when it is dry but still malleable and chewy.

Transfer the fruit leather to a cutting board and cut into twenty 1 x 6-inch (2.5 by 15 cm) strips. Store in an airtight container.

Yield: 20 fruit leathers

Lemony Chia Date Balls

Too much sugar can exacerbate acne and cause breakouts. But that doesn't mean you have to avoid sugar altogether. These zesty no-bake treats are made with a base of protein-rich, heart- and skin-healthy fats from almonds, cashews, and chia seeds, combined with the natural sweetness of fiber-rich dates—no sugar added. Enjoy this satisfying, citrus-infused snack any time you have a sweet craving.

1½ cups (267 g) pitted dates
1   cup (145 g) raw almonds
½   cup (70 g) raw cashews
2   tablespoons (25 g) chia seeds
1   tablespoon (15 ml) freshly squeezed lemon juice
1   teaspoon lemon zest
3   tablespoons (16 g) finely shredded dried coconut

Combine the dates, almonds, cashews, chia seeds, lemon juice, and lemon zest in a food processor and pulse into a coarse and slightly sticky meal. The mixture should stick together when pressed with the fingertips. If it appears too dry, add one or two more dates and process. If it appears too sticky, add a few almonds or cashews and process. Roll the mixture into tablespoon-size (15 g) balls and dredge in the coconut to coat. Store in an airtight container.

Yield: 20 balls

Green Tea & Goji Berry Granola Bars

The antioxidant powers of both green tea and goji berries are great for the skin. In fact, researchers have found that goji berries may help increase antioxidant activity in the skin and minimize the damaging effects that may occur from sun exposure. Combined with omega-3 fatty acid–rich chia seeds and mineral-rich pumpkin seeds, these bars are a treat for the taste buds and the skin.

$^1/_2$ **cup (45 g) dried goji berries**

1 **cup (85 g) shredded dried coconut**

1 **cup (320 g) honey**

$^1/_2$ **cup (73 g) raw almonds, chopped**

$^1/_2$ **cup (32 g) raw pumpkin seeds**

$^1/_4$ **cup (50 g) chia seeds**

1 **tablespoon (16 g) matcha green tea powder**

1 **tablespoon (15 ml) freshly squeezed orange juice**

1 **teaspoon orange zest**

Pinch of sea salt

Placed the dried goji berries in a bowl of warm water for about 5 minutes (just long enough to rehydrate) and then drain thoroughly.

Place all of the ingredients in a large bowl and stir together until thoroughly and evenly combined.

Transfer the mixture to a Teflex-lined dehydrator tray and using a spatula, spread the mixture into an approximately 10-inch (25 cm) square that's $^1/_2$ inch (1 cm) thick. Dehydrate at 105°F (41°C) for about 24 hours until the mixture is dry to the touch on top but still soft.

Remove the tray from the dehydrator and carefully slide the Teflex sheet off of the dehydrator screen. Flip the granola over directly onto the mesh screen and gently peel the Teflex sheet off of the granola. Dehydrate at 105°F (41°C) for another 5 to 6 hours.

Remove the tray from the dehydrator and transfer the square of granola to a dry cutting board. Cut the granola into eight $2^1/_2$ x 5-inch (6 x 13 cm) bars and place the individual bars on the mesh screen, using a spatula to transfer if necessary. Dehydrate the individual bars at 105°F (41°C) for an additional 24 hours. The granola bars are done when they are firm, dry, and slightly chewy.

Yield: 8 bars

Gentle Chia Facial Scrub & Cleanser

This facial scrub was created by Finger Lakes–based Organica Jane, Amy Jane Stewart, a certified holistic aromatherapist and licensed massage therapist (www.organicajane.com). According to Amy, the addition of raw honey is great for cleansing and exfoliating, while the coconut oil works as an antifungal, moisturizing, and age spot–defying cream. You can use the cleanser once or twice a week, although it is gentle enough to use daily.

1   **tablespoon (15 ml) organic coconut oil, melted**
1   **tablespoon (20 g) raw honey**
1   **tablespoon (12.5 g) chia seeds**

Combine all of the ingredients in a small glass jar and mix well with a glass stirrer. Massage well onto the face and neck, avoiding the eyes. Rinse with cool water and pat dry.

Yield: Makes 2 or 3 applications

Note: For additional benefit and to naturally preserve this mixture, add 5 or 6 drops of essential oil. Carrot seed, frankincense, lavender, patchouli, rose, rosewood, and sandalwood are all excellent essential oils for the skin.

Rejuvenating Chia Face Mask

This mask was created by Tricia Marsh, a licensed aesthetician and health coach in upstate New York (www.triciamarsh.com). According to Tricia, this enzymatic mask is ideal for all skin types, helping rid the skin of dead cells and dirt as well as nourishing the skin with essential fatty acids. She notes that the olive oil will calm, soothe, and deeply hydrate the skin, while the bromelain-containing pineapple will help remove dead cells and dirt. Cinnamon acts as a skin disinfectant and revitalizer, while vitamin C–rich lemon helps to tone and refresh the skin. Do a patch test just below the jawline prior to using this mask.

4   **large pineapple chunks or ½ cup (85 g) canned pineapple chunks (organic, BPA-free)**

3   **tablespoons (45 ml) extra-virgin olive oil**

3   **tablespoons (37.5 g) milled chia seeds**

    Juice of ½ lemon

¼   **teaspoon ground cinnamon**

Place all of the ingredients in a blender and blend until almost smooth. Apply a thin layer of the mixture to the face, avoiding the eyes, and leave on for 15 minutes. Rinse with warm water and pat dry. Store in a sealed container (a small mason jar) in the refrigerator for up to 1 month. Bring to room temperature before applying, and be sure to use a clean spatula or hands when reusing to avoid contaminating the mask.

Yield: Makes a scant 1 cup (235 ml)

Note: During the winter months, you can replace the olive oil with raw honey (Tricia's favorite is raw manuka honey) for added moisturizing. You can also use this mask on the elbows, knees, and feet for dry skin.

Soothing Chia Beauty Mask

This chia-based mask was created by Rebecca Casciano, a New York City–based green beauty and wellness coach and makeup artist (www.rebeccacasciano.com). According to Rebecca, the omega-3 fatty acids, phytonutrients, and antioxidants in chia seeds may help soothe inflammation, hydrate the skin, and protect it from free radicals. And adding raw honey, which has antibacterial properties, is helpful for acne, rosacea, and eczema, while anti-inflammatory aloe vera gel can help calm redness, heal scarring, and lessen dark pigmentation.

1   tablespoon (12.5 g) chia seeds
½   cup (120 ml) warm water
1   tablespoon (20 g) raw honey or 1 to 3 teaspoons (5 to 15 g) aloe vera gel (optional)

Combine the chia seeds, warm water, and honey or aloe vera gel and stir well. Let stand for 10 to 15 minutes until thick.

When the mixture turns to a gel, apply 1 to 2 tablespoons (15 to 28 ml) to your face, avoiding the eyes, and leave on for 10 minutes. Rinse with warm water and pat dry. Store in a sealed container (a small mason jar) in the refrigerator.

Yield: Makes a little over ½ cup (120 ml)

CHAPTER 6

Chia Seed Essentials: Tips for Working with Chia

If you have already read through the first five chapters of this book, then you are familiar with some of the incredible ways that adding chia seeds to your diet may help you reach your health goals—from improving digestion and supporting your daily workouts to managing your weight and blood sugars and beautifying your skin. By now, you may have even tried out a few (or many) of the recipes in each chapter and are feeling more inspired than ever to begin working with these super seeds in your kitchen to create your own unique recipes.

In this chapter, I'm going to walk you through the steps of purchasing, storing, and preparing chia seeds in greater detail than previously provided. And with my recipe "templates," you will learn—step by step—how to create endless combinations of chia-based dishes, from chia frescas and puddings to snacks and baked goods. So grab an apron and let's get started!

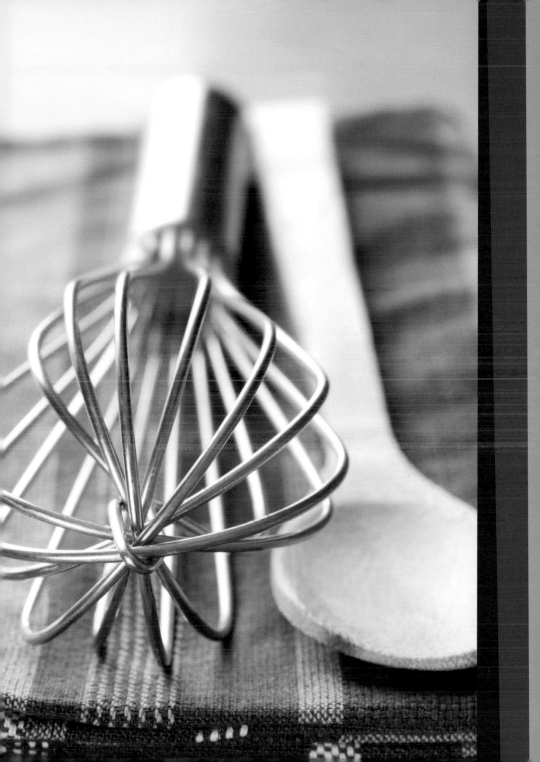

Choosing Chia: Where and What to Buy

Chia seeds are becoming an increasingly popular superfood. Today, you can purchase chia seeds at most supermarkets and health food stores. They are often found in the bulk food section of the market or pre-bagged in the dried fruit and nut or raw food departments. You can also order chia seeds from online retailers. (See the Resources section on page 181 for more information.)

Chia seeds are sold in one of two forms: whole chia seeds or milled chia seeds. Whole chia seeds include both black and white chia seeds, and there is virtually no difference between these seeds from a nutritional and functional standpoint. They can be used interchangeably in any recipe that calls for chia seeds—so which one you choose is simply a matter of personal preference and aesthetics (there are some dishes where white chia seeds will simply look better). Whole chia seeds are typically used to create chia gels, puddings, and frescas; they can be tossed onto salads and into soups and smoothies; and they can be incorporated into an array of dishes (as you may have already discovered and will learn more about here). Milled chia is simply the flour-like chia powder that is created from milling whole chia seeds. Milled chia can also be incorporated into a variety of chia-based dishes, mainly baked goods, where it can be used as a partial flour substitute, but also as a thickener added to soups and smoothies.

Storing Chia: No Refrigeration Necessary

Chia seeds are a rich source of essential fatty acids. But unlike other fat-rich nuts and seeds whose fats may quickly go rancid if not kept refrigerated or frozen, chia seeds can be stored at room temperature. Chia's high antioxidant levels seem to be responsible for protecting their delicate fats and preventing the seed from spoilage. For maximum shelf life, I recommend storing both whole and ground chia seeds in sealed bags or glass jars in a cool, dry location like your kitchen pantry. And be sure to use by the expiration date on the bag.

Chia Prep: Toss and Go

The chia seed is a no-fuss superfood that is incredibly simple to work with. Unlike other seeds (like the pseudograin quinoa), chia seeds do not need to be rinsed or soaked before using. In fact, because the seed will soak up any liquid into which it is placed, I advise against rinsing or soaking unless called for in a recipe. And unlike flaxseeds, which need to be ground in order to access the nutrients within their tough outer shell, chia seeds can be consumed whole—no grinding necessary.

For these reasons, I often think of chia as a "toss-and-go" super seed. You can easily add a spoonful of whole seeds to salads, juices, and smoothies without grinding them. In fact, you can purchase small, single-serving-size packs of chia seeds (or create your own) to stash in your purse or briefcase, allowing you to toss these super seeds into any of your favorite foods and beverages throughout the week and giving your diet a big and convenient boost of nutrients.

Working with Chia: Breaking It Down

Now that you know how to select, store, and prep chia (okay, so there's really no preparation involved), it's time to learn how to begin working with this super seed. In general, whole chia seeds deliver a nice crunch with a very mild (almost undetectable) nut-like flavor—making it a great addition to nearly any food or flavor combination. In this section, I'm going to provide you with a few specific ways to use chia seeds along with a few simple recipes and recipe templates to create your own chia-inspired dishes at home.

Chia Gels

You can start working with chia right away—and take advantage of its valuable nutrients and thickening properties—by making a thick chia gel. Chia gels are created by combining chia seeds with water or juice (preferably 100 percent pure fruit juice) and allowing the mixture to stand until it reaches a thick, gel-like consistency. A few tablespoons (45 to 55 g) of the gel can be eaten alone or tossed into smoothies, soups, dressings, dips, and sauces to help thicken them and provide a boost of the seed's beneficial nutrients. I like to keep a batch of gel in my refrigerator to have on hand any time I need an instant thickener or want to give a dish an immediate nutrient upgrade.

Chia Gel

1   cup (235 ml) water
2   tablespoons plus 1½ teaspoons
     (31 g) chia seeds

Combine the water and chia seeds in a container with a tight-fitting lid (I like to use a mason jar or Pyrex storage dish) and shake to combine. Let the mixture stand for 5 minutes and then shake vigorously to break up any clumps. Let the mixture stand for 20 more minutes, shaking once or twice. The gel is now ready to use, or it can be stored in the refrigerator for 1 to 2 weeks.

Variation: Combine the chia seeds with your favorite super fruit juice (like pure pomegranate, tart cherry, or cranberry) for a sweeter fruit-based gel.

Yield: 1 to 1¼ cups (235 to 295 ml)

Chia Frescas

Chia frescas are beverages that are enjoyed throughout various parts of Mexico, consisting of a mixture of water, lemon or lime juice, sugar, and chia seeds. I personally find chia frescas to be wonderfully refreshing and hydrating, and I love to experiment with a variety of freshly pressed juice combinations (as you may have discovered in the previous chapters) to make my own chia fresca beverages.

Chia Fresca: Step by Step

- Choose 1 cup (235 ml) of your liquid base. Plain water, sparkling water, coconut water, freshly pressed juice (pomegranate and watermelon juices are two of my favorites), or a combination of liquids can form the foundation of your chia fresca.

- Choose 1 tablespoon (15 ml) of your citrus "infusion." A few squeezes of tart and tangy lemon, lime, or grapefruit juice, as well as the sweeter juices of freshly pressed oranges or clementines, will add extra flavor and zest to your liquid base.

- Choose 1 teaspoon of sweetener, more or less to taste. Experiment with the type and amount of sweetener to add to your liquid base, using the smallest amount possible. Raw honey, agave syrup, pure maple syrup, organic cane sugar, or stevia are all good options.

- Optional: Spice up your chia fresca with a small sprinkle of cinnamon, cayenne pepper, grated fresh ginger, or other spice for flavor and nutrition.

- Combine the liquid base, freshly squeezed citrus juice, sweetener, and 1 teaspoon (or more) of chia seeds in a jar with a tight-fitting lid and shake to combine. Let the mixture stand for about 10 minutes, shaking once or twice during that time. Pour into a glass, sprinkle with optional spices, and serve chilled. Refrigerate any unused portion in a sealed container for 2 to 3 days. Serves 1.

Chia Puddings

Chia puddings are thick and creamy puddings similar in texture to tapioca or rice puddings. And with ½ cup (100 g) of chia seeds per batch (enough to yield four ½-cup [225 g]servings), puddings are a great way to get a huge boost of this beneficial seed. Chia puddings are typically created by combining chia seeds in a liquid base of nondairy milk (like almond or coconut milk) or juice and allowing it to thicken. Puddings can be topped with fresh or dried fruits, nuts, seeds, and spices. They are ready to eat in less than 30 minutes, or they can be prepared in the evening and soaked overnight—providing an instant breakfast the following morning.

Chia Pudding: Step by Step

- Choose 2 cups (475 ml) of your liquid base. I find that velvety homemade nut milks (made from almond, cashew, or Brazil nuts) create the creamiest and most delicious bases for chia puddings (see page 141 for instructions on making homemade nut milk). However, you can choose from packaged nondairy milks like unsweetened almond, hemp, or coconut milks, in addition to fruit juices like pomegranate or grape.

- Choose your sweetener. Ideally, use 4 pitted dates or about 1 tablespoon (20 g) of liquid sweetener like raw honey, agave syrup, or pure maple syrup. If you are using fruit juice or sweetened milk as your base, you can omit this step. However, when using packaged nut and seed milks, I recommend choosing unsweetened varieties that you can sweeten naturally to taste. Blending dates with nondairy milk is an incredibly simple and nutritious way to make your pudding base sweeter. But if you are in a rush and have no time to break out the blender, you can use raw honey, agave syrup, or pure maple syrup.

- Choose your "flavor." Add 1 to 2 teaspoons of pure vanilla extract (for vanilla pudding), 1 to 2 tablespoons (6 to 12 g) of raw cacao powder (for chocolate pudding), or 1 tablespoon (8 g) of maca powder (for a caramel-like pudding) for extra flavor.

OVERNIGHT CHIA PUDDING

In Chapter 1, you learned about the important role of breakfast in helping you lose—and keep off—those pesky pounds. If you find that you have little time to prepare this important morning meal, go ahead and make your chia pudding in the evening and let it soak overnight. In the morning, you will have an instant ready-to-eat breakfast for home or on the go—so no excuses for skipping this important first meal of the day. Simply choose any chia pudding recipe in this book and combine all of the ingredients (except the toppings) in a container with a tight-fitting lid. Shake and refrigerate—that's it! In the morning, give the pudding a final shake or stir, pour into a serving bowl, add toppings and sweetener to taste, and serve. It's breakfast made easy!

- To make: Combine your liquid base and sweetener (if using dates to sweeten, blend the dates and liquid in a high-speed blender until smooth), "flavoring," and ½ cup (100 g) chia seeds in a container with a tight-fitting lid and shake. Allow the mixture to rest for 30 minutes, shaking every 5 to 10 minutes. Pour in a serving bowl, add any additional toppings (for example, fresh or dried fruit, nuts, or seeds), and sweeten to taste. Serves 2.

Chia No-Bake Fruit and Nut Bars

For years, clients have consistently asked about the best snacks to help curb hunger and cravings between meals. Fruits and nuts were always (and continue to be) at the top of my list. The combination of natural sugars in fresh and dried fruits with the protein and healthy fats in nuts gives a steady supply of energy to satisfy your body (and your brain). But let's be honest: After a while, a piece of fresh fruit and handful of nuts can get pretty boring. However, I have found that when such simple ingredients are tossed into a food processor to create simple, no-bake fruit and nut bars, they yield some pretty tasty and satisfying combinations of flavors and nutrients that will lift you out of the snacking doldrums. More recently, I've started adding chia seeds to a few of my no-bake bar combinations. Not only do they bump up the fiber and omega-3 fat content of these treats, but they also add a delightful little crunch! You'll be thrilled to come up with some new combinations of snack bars—and ditch the expensive and highly processed energy and sports bars that you may be relying on.

Chia No-Bake Fruit and Nut Bars: Step by Step

- Choose 2 to 2½ cups (300 to 360 g) of your dried fruit base. At least half of this total amount should come from a sticky dried fruit like pitted dates. The other half can consist of any combination of dried fruits, like goji berries, mulberries, cherries, dried apples, raisins, golden raisins, and cranberries.

- Choose 1 to 1½ cups (145 to 220 g) of nuts and seeds. Any combination of almonds, cashews, walnuts, macadamia nuts, Brazil nuts, pumpkin seeds, hemp seeds, flaxseeds, and chia seeds is a good option. When using smaller seeds like hemp, flax, and chia, I recommend using a maximum of ½ cup of these seeds, with the remaining amount coming from nuts and larger seeds like sunflower and pumpkin.

- To make: Line a cutting board with waxed paper. Combine all of the ingredients in a food processor and process into a coarse "dough." The dough should stick together when pressed with the fingertips. If the dough appears too dry, add one or two more dates and process. If it appears too sticky, add a few nuts or a small scoop of chia seeds and process. Transfer the dough to the cutting board. Press the dough into a large ball and place on the waxed paper in the center of the cutting board. Place a second sheet of waxed paper on top of the dough and flatten with the palm of your hand. Using a rolling pin, roll the dough out (with the waxed paper on top) into a ½-inch-thick (1 cm) rectangle, trimming the edges of the dough if needed. Cut the dough into twelve 1 x 3-inch (2.5 x 7.5 cm) bars—or any size or shape of your choosing.

Baking with Chia

Chia is great for baking. You can use whole chia seeds as an egg replacer (see below), toss whole chia seeds into batter, or use milled chia seeds as a partial flour substitute in your favorite traditional baked recipes. As a general rule, I have found that you can substitute up to one-quarter of the flour in your recipe with milled chia seeds. So if your recipe calls for 2 cups (250 g) of flour, you can likely use ¼ cup (50 g) of milled chia seeds and 1¾ cups (219 g) of traditional flour. Because of its rich fiber content, you can expect the texture of your chia-enriched baked goods to be slightly denser—and they may also take slightly longer to bake (3 to 5 minutes more). Just be sure to insert a toothpick into the center of your baked good, which should come out clean when done. And because chia adds to the density of baked goods, I recommend using chia as either an egg replacer or a flour alternative in baking—not both. As you will notice in this chapter, I typically choose to use chia as an egg replacer (using all gluten-free flour) or as a partial flour substitute (using an egg or two) in baked goods.

When choosing milled chia seeds, you can choose either white milled seeds or regular milled seeds—the only difference being color. When I add milled chia to baked goods, I tend to use the traditional milled seeds. But when I add milled chia as a thickener to creamy and light-colored soups, I prefer using the white

INSTANT EGG SUBSTITUTE

Chia seeds can be mixed with water to create a super-thick gel that can be used as an egg substitute, which is a great alternative for vegans or those with an egg allergy. To make your own chia-based egg substitute, simply whisk together 1 tablespoon (12.5 g) of chia seeds with 3 tablespoons (45 ml) of water for each large egg. Allow the mixture to stand for about 15 minutes until thick and then incorporate into your recipe as you would an egg. It's so easy!

milled chia to prevent any color changes in my soups. But functionally and nutritionally, both milled varieties are the same. Note that some manufacturers also sell a "gluten-free chia flour," which is often a blend of milled chia seeds and brown rice or other flours. In this case, the chia flour can be substituted cup for cup with the traditional flour. However, be sure to consult the package instructions or manufacturer's Web site, as usage may vary among brands.

Recipes At A Glance

Chia-Inspired Baked Goods

Chunky Chewy Oatmeal & Raisin Cookies

According to my family and friends, you can't tell the difference between these gluten-free, chia-enriched cookies and the traditional version.

½ cup (68 g) Bob's Red Mill all-purpose gluten-free baking flour

2 tablespoons (25 g) milled chia seeds

½ teaspoon baking soda

½ teaspoon xanthan gum

¼ teaspoon sea salt

½ cup (1 stick, or 112 g) butter, softened

¾ cup (170 g) lightly packed brown sugar

1 large egg

½ teaspoon pure vanilla extract

1½ cups (120 g) rolled oats

¾ cup (110 g) raisins

Preheat the oven to 350°F (180°C, or gas mark 4). Line 2 baking sheets with parchment paper.

In a small bowl, stir together the flour, milled chia seeds, baking soda, xanthan gum, and sea salt. Using an electric mixer, beat together the butter and brown sugar. Beat in the egg and vanilla extract. On low speed, beat in the dry ingredients. Using a spatula, fold in the oats and raisins.

Drop about 2 tablespoons (28 g) of cookie dough per cookie (I use a #40 scoop) onto the baking sheets and bake until golden brown, 12 to 15 minutes. Let stand on the sheets for a few minutes before transferring to a wire cooling rack. Store in an airtight container.

Yield: About 20 cookies

Crumb-Top Coffee Cake Muffins

This muffin is a modified version of my aunt's quick coffee cake. In this recipe, I combine ¼ cup (50 g) of milled chia with gluten-free baking flour. The batter becomes incredibly dense while mixing, but it yields a nicely textured muffin.

For the muffins:

1¼ cups (170 g) Bob's Red Mill all-purpose, gluten-free baking flour

¾ cup (150 g) sugar

¼ cup (50 g) milled chia seeds

2 teaspoons baking powder

1½ teaspoons xanthan gum

½ teaspoon salt

½ cup (1 stick, or 112 g) butter, softened

1 large egg

½ cup (120 ml) milk (nondairy or regular)

For the topping:

½ cup (50 g) raw walnuts, chopped

¼ cup (60 g) brown sugar

1 tablespoon (7 g) finely ground almond meal/flour

1 tablespoon (14 g) butter, melted

1 teaspoon ground cinnamon

Preheat the oven to 375°F (190°C, or gas mark 5). Lightly oil 10 cups of a muffin pan or line with paper cupcake liners.

To make the muffins: In a small bowl, combine the flour, sugar, milled chia seeds, baking powder, xanthan gum, and salt. In a large bowl, whisk together the butter, egg, and milk. Stir in the dry ingredients and mix until just combined (the batter will be very dense and thick). Using a spatula, fill the cups about three-quarters full of batter.

To make the topping: Mix together all of the ingredients. Sprinkle 1 tablespoon (15 g) of topping onto each muffin. Bake for 25 to 30 minutes until golden brown on top and a toothpick inserted comes out clean. Transfer to a wire cooling rack to cool.

Yield: 10 muffins

Peach & Black Raspberry Cobbler

In this fall favorite, I use milled chia seeds in place of corn or potato starch to help thicken the sweet and rich fruit filling. A combination of gluten-free flour and delicate almond meal (rather than the denser milled chia) makes a perfect topping for this cobbler.

For the filling:

3   cups (510 g) peeled and sliced fresh peaches (or [750 g] thawed frozen)

2   cups (250 g) fresh black raspberries (or [500 g] thawed frozen)

1/2 cup (100 g) sugar

1/4 cup (50 g) milled chia seeds

1   teaspoon freshly squeezed lemon juice

For the topping:

1/2 cup (68 g) Bob's Red Mill all-purpose gluten-free flour

1/2 cup (56 g) finely ground almond meal/flour

1   tablespoon (13 g) sugar

1 1/2 teaspoons baking powder

1/2 teaspoon salt

1/4 teaspoon ground cinnamon

1/2 cup (120 ml) milk (nondairy or regular)

3   tablespoons (42 g) butter, softened

1   tablespoon (15 g) brown sugar

Preheat the oven to 400°F (200°C, or gas mark 6).

To make the filling: Toss the peaches and berries with the sugar, chia seeds, and lemon juice in a large saucepan. Cook over medium-high heat, stirring occasionally, until the mixture thickens and begins to boil. Once boiling, cook and stir for an additional 1 minute. Remove from the heat and pour into an ungreased 2-quart (1.9 L) casserole dish.

To make the topping: Combine the flour, almond meal, sugar, baking powder, salt, and cinnamon in a bowl. Add the milk and butter and mix by hand until it thickens. Drop the dough by the tablespoon (15 g) onto the fruit. Sprinkle the brown sugar on the drops of dough. Bake for 20 to 25 minutes until the topping is browned. Let stand for at least 10 minutes to thicken and cool slightly. Serve warm.

Yield: Serves 4 to 6

Blueberry Buckle

This is a greatly modified version of my mom's traditional blueberry buckle, which I frequently enjoyed during childhood summers after our blueberry-picking excursions. In this recipe, I use chia as an egg replacer. The result is a very thick and dense batter that bakes into a nicely textured cake with a sweet and crumbly topping. To make this recipe vegan, simply substitute coconut oil or a nondairy butter substitute (like Earth Balance) for the butter.

For the filling:

1   tablespoon (12.5 g) chia seeds

3   tablespoons (45 ml) water

2   cups (272 g) Bob's Red Mill all-purpose gluten-free baking flour

2   teaspoons baking powder

2   teaspoons xanthan gum

1/2   teaspoon salt

1/4   cup (1/2 stick, or 55 g) butter, softened

3/4   cup (150 g) sugar

3/4   cup (175 ml) milk (nondairy or regular)

2   cups (290 g) fresh blueberries

For the topping:

1/2   cup (100 g) sugar

1/3   cup (37 g) finely ground almond meal/flour

1/2   teaspoon ground cinnamon

1/4   cup (1/2 stick, or 55 g) butter, softened

Preheat the oven to 350°F (180°C, or gas mark 4). Lightly oil a 9-inch (23 cm) square baking dish. (I like to use an organic canola oil spray.)

To make the filling: Whisk together the chia seeds and water and set aside to thicken to make the egg replacer. In a small bowl, combine the flour, baking powder, xanthan gum, and salt. Using an electric mixer, beat together the butter, sugar, and chia egg replacer. Stir in the milk. Stir in the dry ingredients. Fold in the blueberries (the batter will be very thick). Spread the batter into the baking dish.

To make the topping: Mix together the sugar, almond meal, cinnamon, and butter. Sprinkle the topping over the cake.

Bake for 45 to 50 minutes until a toothpick inserted in the center comes out clean. Let cool completely in the pan before cutting and serving.

Yield: Serves 9

Broccoli & Cheese Chia Puffs

These hearty, muffin-like "puffs" make a great appetizer, side dish, or snack. In this recipe, I incorporate milled chia seeds into a gluten-free batter.

2   **cups (142 g) broccoli florets**

1³/₄ **cups (238 g) Bob's Red Mill all-purpose gluten-free baking flour**

¹/₄   **cup (50 g) milled chia seeds**

2   **teaspoons baking powder**

¹/₂   **teaspoon salt**

2   **cups (475 ml) milk**

2   **large eggs**

2   **cups (225 g) shredded Cheddar cheese**

¹/₂   **cup (50 g) grated Parmesan cheese**

Preheat the oven to 350°F (180°C, or gas mark 4). Lightly oil 12 to 14 cups of a muffin pan or pans. (I like to use an organic canola oil spray.)

Steam the broccoli until bright green and crisp-tender, about 5 minutes. Rinse under cold water, drain, and chop. In a small bowl, stir together the flour, milled chia seeds, baking powder, and salt. In a large bowl, whisk together the milk and eggs. Add the dry ingredients to the wet ingredients and stir together until just combined. Fold in the cheeses and broccoli.

Pour ¹/₃ cup (80 ml) of batter into each muffin cup. Bake for 35 to 40 minutes until a toothpick inserted into a muffin puff comes out clean. Let stand in the pan for a few minutes to cool before transferring the puffs to a wire cooling rack.

Yield: 12 to 14 puffs

Where can I buy chia seeds?

You can purchase whole and milled chia seeds at most supermarkets and health food stores. If your local market does not carry chia seeds, you can order through one of the online retailers listed in the Resources section (page 181).

What is the difference between black and white chia seeds?

There is virtually no difference between black and white chia seeds from either a nutritional or a functional standpoint. The only difference between the two seeds is their color, so use of either is simply a matter of personal preference.

Should chia seeds be stored in the refrigerator?

Due to their high levels of antioxidants, chia seeds do not need to be refrigerated or frozen. They can be stored in an airtight container at room temperature. Just be sure to use them by the expiration date listed on the package to ensure optimal freshness.

Do I need to grind chia seeds before eating?

No, unlike flaxseeds, chia seeds do not need to be ground before eating in order to access their beneficial nutrients. You can eat these crunchy seeds whole or milled.

Are the chia seeds I eat the same as chia seeds sold with the popular Chia Pets?

The chia seeds that you eat are essentially the same as those sold with the popular Chia Pets—but those sold with Chia Pets should not be consumed. You should only eat chia seeds that are labeled and sold for consumption, not those used as part of a household decoration.

How much chia should I eat each day?

Chia is a whole food, not a supplement, so there are no specific "dosages" that you need to consume each day. The amount of chia you should consume is highly individual. Most manufacturers list serving sizes as 1 tablespoon (12.5 g), which provides about 4.5 grams of fiber and 2.5 grams of omega-3 fatty acids. And in research studies, the safety of chia seed consumption has been demonstrated in quantities up to 31 to 38.5 grams (2½ to 3¼ tablespoons) per day. Some people, particularly those looking to boost the content of omega-3 fatty acids in their diet, may benefit from as a little as a teaspoon or two of chia seeds daily, while those looking to boost their fiber intake may benefit from an additional 2 to 3 tablespoons (25 to 37.5 g) of chia seeds daily. As you begin to add chia seeds to your diet, listen to your body; you may find that you do not require as much as you might have thought. A few teaspoons (rather than tablespoons) may be all you need to keep your digestive tract moving, give you the energy to sustain a long workout, or meet another health goal.

Is it possible to eat too much chia?
It is possible to eat too much of nearly any food—even unprocessed whole foods. I don't recommend consuming more than 2 to 3 tablespoons (25 to 37.5 g) of chia seeds per day due to their high fiber content. Even though amounts slightly higher than that may be safe, there is no evidence to show that consuming more offers any additional benefits to health.

Are there any side effects from eating chia?
No significant adverse effects from consuming chia seeds have been reported in any research studies to date. However, the participants of one clinical trial did report gastrointestinal side effects. Consuming high-fiber foods like chia—especially consuming too much, too soon, and without increasing fluid intake—may cause stomach cramping, bloating, and abdominal discomfort. To minimize potential discomfort, be sure to add chia seeds gradually to your diet—perhaps a teaspoon at a time—especially if you have been eating a low-fiber diet. Spreading your chia intake out over the course of a day—a teaspoon here or there rather than a tablespoon at one time—may also prevent stomach upset. In addition, be sure to drink plenty of water. As you increase the fiber in your diet, your body will require extra fluids to keep that fiber moving through your digestive tract.

Is there anyone who should not consume chia?

Consuming chia seeds may not be advised for individuals with undiagnosed gastro-intestinal disorders. As mentioned in Chapter 3, if you are suffering from chronic or acute gastrointestinal issues, you should be evaluated by your health care provider before making any drastic changes to your diet. Adding a fiber-rich food like chia to the diet may worsen symptoms in some people. In addition, chia seeds may not be advised for those with hypotension (low blood pressure), as they may further lower blood pressure levels in some individuals. Please consult your health care provider if you are unsure whether or not to add chia seeds to your diet.

I am a vegan. Can I use chia egg replacer in any baked good recipes that call for eggs?

Yes, absolutely! Chia is great for baking and Chia Egg Replacer (page 171) can be used in nearly any baked good recipe that calls for eggs. However, it is important to note that I rarely use both milled chia seeds and chia egg replacer in the same recipe, as the final product tends to be very dense (and there are a few baked good recipes in this book that incorporate both whole eggs and milled chia). To make those recipes vegan, you can substitute a vegan egg replacer (like Ener-G egg replacer) for the eggs. Or you can create a Chia Egg Replacer and omit the milled chia seeds, instead adding an equivalent amount of flour in place of the milled chia seeds. Substitute a nondairy butter substitute (such as Earth Balance) for the butter in a 1:1 ratio. Your choice!

Chia: Highlights of the Ultimate Super Seed

- Whole food—not a supplement
- Naturally gluten-free
- Antioxidant rich—can be stored at room temperature without spoiling
- No grinding necessary—enjoy whole or milled seeds for a nutrient boost
- Mildly nutty, almost neutral taste—perfect addition to nearly any dish
- Easy to use—simply toss into your favorite foods and beverages

1 ounce of chia seeds contains:*
- Nearly 10 grams of dietary fiber—the amount in a large head of lettuce
- Nearly 5 grams of protein—the amount in a small egg
- 179 milligrams of calcium—more than the amount in 1/2 cup (120 ml) of whole milk
- More than 2 grams of iron—the amount in nearly 3 cups (60 grams) of fresh spinach
- More omega-3 fatty acids than an equivalent serving of flaxseeds
- More magnesium than an equivalent serving of peanuts

*1 ounce (28.35 g) is equivalent to about 2 to 2½ tablespoons of chia seeds.

SOURCE: USDA NATIONAL NUTRIENT DATABASE FOR STANDARD REFERENCE, RELEASE 25. HTTP://NDB.NAL.USDA.GOV/

Chia seeds can be found in most supermarkets and health food stores. You can also purchase them online through a number of retailers.

AZChia Products	www.azchia.com
Barlean's Organic Oils	www.barleans.com
Bob's Red Mill	www.bobsredmill.com
Foods Alive	www.foodsalive.com
Green Plus	www.greensplus.com
Living Intentions	www.shop.livingintentions.com
Navitas Naturals	www.navitasnaturals.com
NOW Foods	www.nowfoods.com
Nutiva	www.nutiva.com
Spectrum	www.spectrumorganics.com
Sunfood	www.sunfood.com
The Chia Co	www.thechiaco.com.au
TruRoots	www.truroots.com

With gratitude...

To the loves of my life, Gary and Maria, for your unconditional love and endless support. You make my heart smile and my soul sing. I will love you forever and always, to infinity and beyond.

To my parents who continue to support my work, especially my dad who has always encouraged me to follow my dreams, and my mom for decades of incredible meals and open access to her recipe box.

To my beautiful friends, especially Gabrielle, Jen G, Jen K, Katie, Kristin, and Trish. I am truly grateful to be in the company of such a wonderful group of strong, smart, and kind women—and honored to call you all my friends.

To my go-to green beauty experts, Amy Jane Stewart, Rebecca Casciano, and Tricia Marsh. Thank you for your contributions to this book and for sharing your wisdom that undoubtedly helps women glow inside and out.

To the amazing team at Fair Winds Press, including Jill Alexander, John Gettings, Renae Haines, Heather Godin, Paul Burgess, Kathie Alexander, Glenn Scott, Catrine Kelty, Valerie Cimino, Marilyn Kecyk, Katie Fawkes, and Dalyn Miller. Your synchronized efforts have brought the text and recipes in each book to life so that those who read may be inspired. You are a dream team and I thank you.

Lauri Boone, R.D., is a registered dietitian, speaker, writer, and author of *Powerful Plant-Based Superfoods* (Fair Winds Press, 2013). A member of Dietitians in Integrative and Functional Medicine and graduate of the Institute for Integrative Nutrition, Lauri has a passion for good food and clean eating and emphasizes a whole foods, holistic approach to health and wellness. She has contributed to numerous print and online publications and blogs including *One Green Planet, The Pilates Forum,* and *The Wise Mom.* She has also appeared in several media outlets including *The Huffington Post, The Daily Messenger* ("Dietitian Touts Alternative Nutrition"), CBS Affiliate WROC-8, CNN, NBC 10's Roc City Tonight, BBC Radio, and more. A health and wellness expert on ChickRx and Learn it Live, Lauri offers nutrition advice and instructs online food and nutrition classes for students around the world. She resides in the beautiful Finger Lakes region of upstate New York with her family.